Health Care Ethics Committees

The Next Generation

Judith Wilson Ross, M.A.

John W. Glaser, S.T.D.

Dorothy Rasinski-Gregory, J.D., M.D.

Joan McIver Gibson, Ph.D.

Corrine Bayley, M.A.

AHA books are published by
American Hospital Publishing, Inc.,
an American Hospital Association company

The views expressed in this publication are strictly those of the authors and do not necessarily represent official positions of the American Hospital Association.

Library of Congress Cataloging-in-Publication Data

Health care ethics committees : the next generation / Judith Wilson
   Ross . . . [et al.].
       p.   cm.
   Includes bibliographical references.
   ISBN 1-55648-103-9 (pbk.)
   1. Ethics committees. 2. Medical ethics. I. Ross, Judith
Wilson.
   [DNLM: 1. Ethics Committees—organization & administration.
WX 159 H4335 1993]
R725.3.H43   1993
174'.2—dc20
DNLM/DLC
for Library of Congress   93-17509
                                                        CIP

Catalog no. 058300

©1993 by American Hospital Publishing, Inc.,
an American Hospital Association company

Printed in the USA

AHA is a service mark of the American Hospital Association used under license by American Hospital Publishing, Inc.

Text set in Times Roman
4M—8/93—0348

Audrey Kaufman, Acquisitions/Development Editor
Anne Hermann, Production Editor
Peggy DuMais, Production Coordinator
Cheryl Kusek, Cover Designer
Marcia Bottoms, Books Division Assistant Director
Brian Schenk, Books Division Director

Contents

List of Figures

About the Authors

Corrine Bayley, M.A., is vice-president for ethics and corporate values at St. Joseph Health System in Orange, California. She is also on the staff of the system's Center for Healthcare Ethics. Her past experience includes seven years as a hospital chief executive officer. Ms. Bayley is a fellow of The Hastings Center, a consultant to nine ethics committees, and a lecturer in the Department of Medicine at the University of California at Irvine. She is cofounder and a board member of California Health Decisions, an innovative grass-roots organization whose mission is to educate and involve the public in ethical issues and health care. Ms. Bayley has published several articles and book chapters and is coauthor of *Handbook for Hospital Ethics Committees* (Chicago: American Hospital Publishing, 1986).

Joan McIver Gibson, Ph.D., is director of the Center for Health Law and Ethics, Institute of Public Law at the University of New Mexico (in Albuquerque), where she is currently focusing her research and teaching efforts on the Values History Form (which she developed), mediation and medical ethics, and the role of the state and federal judiciary in bioethics issues. Since 1982, Dr. Gibson has also chaired the St. Joseph Healthcare System Medical Ethics Committee, also located in Albuquerque. She has taught ethics, with a special emphasis on health care, at the undergraduate level as well as in graduate medical, law, and nursing schools.

John W. Glaser, S.T.D., is currently assistant vice-president of St. Joseph Health System in Orange, California, and director of the system's Center for Healthcare Ethics. Previously, Mr. Glaser was director of the Ethics Program, Sisters of Mercy Health Corporation in Farmington Hills, Michigan, and assistant professor of religious studies at the University of Detroit.

Dorothy Rasinski-Gregory, J.D., M.D., is an associate in the Center for Healthcare Ethics at St. Joseph Health System in Orange, California. She is also a private consultant in legal medicine and risk management. Dr. Rasinski-Gregory was previously adjunct professor of medicine at the University of California at Irvine; past president of the American College of Legal Medicine headquartered in Milwaukee, Wisconsin; and associate chief of staff for education at the Long Beach VA Hospital, where she established and chaired the ethics committee. She serves on the editorial boards of the *Journal of Legal Medicine,* the *Cambridge Quarterly of Healthcare Ethics,* and the *Journal of Clinical Ethics.*

Judith Wilson Ross, M.A., is an associate at the Center for Healthcare Ethics at St. Joseph Health System in Orange, California. Originally trained in English literature, she has been writing about and teaching bioethics since 1977. She has taught at UCLA in the College of Letters and Sciences, the School of Law, and the School of Medicine (in the positions of associate director of the Program in Medical Ethics, assistant professor of medicine, and assistant director of the Program in Medicine, Law, and Human Values). In addition, Ms. Ross has worked extensively with ethics committees in public, private, and teaching hospitals, as well as in health maintenance organizations.

Ms. Ross is coeditor of the *HEC Forum;* editor of *Ethical Currents;* editor of *Healthcare Ethics Literature Review;* and editor of the bimonthly *Western Bioethics Network,* a collaborative newsletter of the Center for Healthcare Ethics (Orange, California) and the Pacific Center for Health Policy and Ethics (University of Southern California). The author of many articles and reviews on patient care and health policy issues, she is coauthor (with William Winslade) of *Choosing Life and Death: A Guide for Patients, Families, and Professionals* (New York City: The Free Press, 1986) and *The Insanity Plea: The Uses and Abuses of the Insanity Defense* (New York City: Scribner's, 1983) and the principal author of *A Handbook for Hospital Ethics Committees* (Chicago: American Hospital Publishing, 1986).

Preface

Interest in and support for ethics committees continue to grow in the United States, as well as in Canada, Europe, and Japan. Many nursing and medical professional organizations have endorsed them, as have various governmental commissions, hospital associations, and advocacy groups. Maryland has mandated their establishment in that state; New York has proposed legislation giving them extensive statutory authority; and California has passed new legislation requiring the creation of multidisciplinary committees to review treatment decisions for incapacitated patients without surrogates who reside in long-term care facilities. The Joint Commission on Accreditation of Healthcare Organizations' (JCAHO's) 1992 standards include a new requirement for a forum to resolve ethical issues and suggest that creation of an ethics committee would be one way to satisfy this requirement. Two new journals for ethics committee members have come into being: the *HEC [HealthCare Ethics Committee] Forum,* now in its fifth year, and the *Cambridge Quarterly of Healthcare Ethics,* now in its second year. The third annual national conference for ethics committees, sponsored by the International Bioethics Institute, was held in the spring of 1993. Thus, 17 years after the New Jersey Supreme Court's discussion of ethics committees in the *Quinlan* decision,[1] it appears that the idea of multidisciplinary committees in which ethical problems in health care can be addressed has survived and flourished.

However, more than just the idea has flourished. The actual number of committees continues to grow. A survey conducted for the President's Commission's 1983 volume *Deciding to Forego Life-Sustaining Treatment* reported that fewer than 1 percent of hospitals had ethics committees involved in patient decision making.[2] By 1985, surveys were reporting that 50 percent of hospitals in the United States had ethics committees.[3] Currently, the estimate is around 60 percent, although a national survey has not been conducted for some years. State and regional networks of ethics committees have done some surveys of their own areas, and these surveys suggest that a 65 to 85 percent figure is possible.[4] It is not unlikely that in the very near future, all hospitals and many long-term care facilities will have ethics committees.

With all this success, is there a need for a book on creating an effective ethics committee? We think so. Advocating the potential value of an ethics committee is not the same as creating a viable, effective, lively, cohesive, and "ethical" ethics committee—one that is committed to moral community. In a provocative article on feminist medical ethics, Virginia Warren has written about the tendency of the bioethics field to concentrate solely on what she calls "crisis issues" (transplantation, forgoing treatment, and so on), and largely to ignore what she ironically calls "housekeeping issues" (for example, the problematic hierarchy in physician–nurse relationships, getting physicians to talk to patients about advance directives, and so on).[5]

The same phenomenon is seen in ethics committees. For example, there is often intense interest whether a hospital lawyer should be on the ethics committee, but little discussion of his or her function on the committee. Similarly, there is often great interest in whether the committee should be organized as a medical staff committee or an administrative committee but little thought given to how the choice affects the committee's ongoing operations. (For example, in some institutions an ethics committee organized as a medical staff committee may not begin its meeting until a quorum *not of members but of physicians* is present. The message this sends to nonphysician members is rarely noted, but it undoubtedly has an impact on the committee's effectiveness.)

Warren differentiates *crisis issues* from *housekeeping issues* in several ways, including their temporal nature: Crisis issues are resolved at some point in time; housekeeping issues go on and on. If ethics committees are to thrive and contribute to their institution's understanding of itself as a moral community, they will have to pay more attention to the housekeeping issues, to the dailiness of ethics committee life. In this book we delineate these issues and suggest strategies for dealing with them. In addition, we have observed three other troubling factors: support for the committee's sense of mission, enthusiasm for the committee's objectives, and definition of the committee's goals.

First, support for ethics committees has largely been support in principle only, with little practical help or guidance from the institutions themselves. This means that committees are sometimes formed at the order of the chief executive officer or the medical staff executive committee, but then are not given a meaningful role or helped to find one. Such committees are likely to exist in name only or to become institutional window dressing. They are very much in need of help to either restore their sense of mission or find the mission that previously eluded them. This book provides help in creating a committee that has a sense of community and that can formulate a reasonable mission, which is the first but not the only step in developing a successful ethics committee.

Second, support for the *idea* of ethics committees does not necessarily translate into enthusiasm for them. Consequently, committees are sometimes created and then find themselves the object of specific or general disapproval. Ethicists and health care professionals (and perhaps the lay public) often doubt the value of this innovation. Within the field of bioethics itself, endorsement of ethics committees is ambiguous at best and sometimes hostile, especially with respect to whether clinical ethics consultants or ethics committees can best serve the institution's needs. Despite organized medicine's endorsement of ethics committees, many physicians seem unsympathetic or even hostile to them, perhaps because they feel the existence of an ethics committee implies the institution's reluctance to trust them to make treatment decisions without some kind of oversight.[6] Nurses, too, have sometimes been dubious about the value of ethics committees with their long discussions, a process that one nurse described as "agonizing by committee."[7]

It is difficult to know what the lay public knows or thinks about ethics committees. One early survey (1984) found that, at least in theory, three-fourths of patients thought ethics committees were a good idea, although few actually knew of the existence of such a committee.[8] Certainly patients seldom seek an ethics committee's assistance, even when they are informed that one exists. In the media, ethics committees are likely to be characterized as the "bad guys" (or at least the "incompetent guys"). For example, one television movie, *Baby Girl Scott,* tells the story of the parents of a seriously ill newborn who try to get the physicians to stop treatment and let their very prematurely born infant die. After the ethics committee meets to discuss the issue with the health care team (the parents are not allowed to attend), the couple is told by a kindly but apologetic woman that their plea to stop treatment has failed. "Ethics committees," she says, "are not noted for their courage." She tells the couple this by way of explaining the committee's failure to side with the family against the obviously bad-guy physician. Doubtless, more Americans have heard this line than have seen any of the guidelines and articles asserting the value of ethics committees. Thus, patients also may be ambivalent about ethics committees, hoping the committees will help them but unsure whom the committees are really trying to protect.

Committees that feel unwelcome in their institutions often want to reach out to patients and their health professional colleagues but are uncertain about how to do so. Gaining credibility and proving the committee's value are not easy in a hostile or doubtful environment. It is even more difficult for a committee that is unsure about what it stands for and whom it represents. This book will help committees to better understand the scope of their task and ways to achieve it that can persuade rather than alienate others in the institution.

Third, experienced ethics committees frequently lose their momentum and members suffer a loss of morale after having credibly performed education, policy writing, and case review for several years. With few case consultation requests and forgoing treatment policies already written, such committees become uncertain about what to do other than to meet monthly and talk to one another. "What should we be doing?" these committee members ask. Although the answer must come from within their own institutional setting, this book can help frame the questions these committee members need to ask and will suggest some routes to follow once they have chosen a goal.

This is a time of regrouping for ethics committees. The first flush of enthusiasm generated by the articles, conferences, discussions, and court decisions about forgoing treatment conflicts has passed, even if problematic cases still occur. Do-not-resuscitate policies have been agreed on, even if practice is not always consistent with policy and more education is needed. Patients are now routinely informed about their rights to consent to and to refuse treatment and their right to make advance directives, even if most do not. The passage of the Patient Self-Determination Act marks the end of the first phase of ethics committees.

In the first phase, a consensus was reached that related largely to decisions about life-sustaining treatment. Despite the narrow focus of this discussion, the larger message was that health care involved values and that values needed to be taken seriously. The proliferation of articles on ethics in health care testifies to the fact that both health care professionals and health care institutions have been alerted to the importance of ethical sensitivity in their practice. The task of ethics committees in this second phase is to keep that sense of importance alive, not only with respect to forgoing treatment but also to all the decisions and practices that make the experience of health care a critical factor in human life. The task is difficult and the time available to committees is limited, so committee work needs to be planned carefully.

Ethics committees differ from each other, even if they all have the same name. Although little has been published about them, there is an opportunity to share what information exists. In this book, we use the existing quantitative information, but we also rely largely on our combined experiences with the ethics committees with which we work and of which we are members, as well as on information and experiences that so many ethics committee members have generously shared with us at conferences and workshops and through newsletters. In this way, we hope to enhance the sharing of information among ethics committees across the country as each works to make a difference in its own institution and community.

The material in this book is divided into 12 chapters beginning with the discussion in *chapter 1* of the origins of ethics committees and how this history has led to confusion about the nature of ethics committees. This chapter also describes some current trends in the field.

Chapter 2 provides a list of activities and projects that ethics committees might consider undertaking to expand their sense of the scope of appropriate work for ethics committees.

Chapter 3 describes the current disagreements about ethical theory in applied bioethics that frequently lead members to feel that they either do not know enough about ethics or have heard too much that makes no sense. It also discusses why it is important to have some understanding of these disagreements.

Chapter 4 looks at both the content and the process of the monthly ethics committee meeting to help make meetings more efficient, productive, and involving for the members.

Chapter 5 presents a variety of methods for conducting education for committee members and suggests some basic levels of knowledge they should have.

Chapter 6 discusses how committees might think about whether and when to write policies and how to go about the process of policy writing in ways that will not bog the committee down.

Chapter 7 presents more and less effective ways of doing case consultation and explores means of sidestepping some of the controversial aspects of this function.

Chapter 8 analyzes the reasons for evaluation and the various forms evaluation can take, and provides committees with techniques and instruments to begin evaluating their own committee process.

Chapter 9 looks at the role of lawyers on ethics committees and highlights liability concerns for ethics committee members: how to stay out of litigation and how to appropriately protect members should the committee become involved in litigation.

Chapter 10 considers a number of issues involved in the successful operation of a committee—the relationships of ethics committees with ethics consultants and clinical ethicists, the practice of rotating memberships, the role of former chairpersons, and the relationships between the ethics committee and other committees that also have responsibility for ethical practice in the institution.

Chapter 11 probes the differences between ethics committees in acute care and non-acute care institutions. These differences should lead to ethics committees in long-term care that are quite different from those in acute care, in both their membership and their mission. Acute care ethics committees may be of help to long-term care facilities, but they need to understand the differences between the issues in the two settings.

Chapter 12 speculates about the future of ethics committees and advocates a role for them that is broader than is often imagined or argued, as well as is less involved in individual patient care decisions.

Most of the chapters include activities, exercises, and questions to help committee members think about a particular issue or committee process. We believe that ethics committees work best when they are living out the democratic impulse that led to their creation. This means that all members have to participate, feel involved, and believe that their presence and their contribution will make a difference. If there is a single thing that can be said of ethics committees, it is that their members want ethical concerns to be important to their institution and to have that importance demonstrated. The ethics committee itself should be the first place where those values are lived out.

Notes and References

1. *In the matter of Karen Quinlan.* 70 N.J. 10, 1976.

2. *Deciding to Forego Life-Sustaining Treatment, The President's Commission for the Study of Ethical Problems in Medicine and Biomedical and Behavioral Research.* Washington, DC: U.S. Government Printing Office, 1983.

3. Ethics committees double since 83: survey. *Hospitals* 59(21):6–64, 1985.

4. Personal communications: Daniel Lang (Los Angeles Committee Task Force), June 1991; Myra Christopher (Mid-West Bioethics Center), July 1991; and Evelyn Van Allen (Minnesota Ethics Committee Network), July 1991.

5. Warren, V. L. Feminist directions in medical ethics. *Hypatia* 4(2):73–87, 1989; reprinted in *HEC Forum* 4(1):19–36, 1992.

6. This is the general thesis of David Rothman's *Strangers at the Bedside.* New York City: Basic Books, 1991.

7. Tisdale, S. Swept away by technology. *American Journal of Nursing* 86(4):429–30, Apr. 1986.

8. Youngner, S. J., Coulton, C., Juknialis, B. W., and Jackson, D. L. Patients' attitudes toward hospital ethics committees. *Law, Medicine, and Health Care* 12(1):21–25, 1984.

Acknowledgments

We wish to extend our thanks to the many people who helped us throughout the course of developing this book:

To Don Phillips, Carol Stocking, Evelyn Van Allen, Phillip Foubert, Ronald B. Miller, Robert L. Schwartz, David Blake, Vicki Michel, Sharon Mass, Foster Mobley, and Anna Kaufman, whose thoughts on various topics were of great help. We hope we have used those thoughts wisely; if there are misjudgments, they are surely ours, not theirs.

To Lauri Rogers and Jennifer Dodos, who helped us keep track of and move around the many versions of each chapter, coping with problems that only those who have worked with electronic information and coauthors in different states and countries can imagine.

To St. Joseph Health System, which generously supported the planning and execution of this book.

To our editor, Audrey Kaufman, who helped us gracefully and judiciously through a project that took longer than she or we had anticipated.

And to the many ethics committee members we have known and worked with over the years, and especially to the members of the health care institution bioethics committees to which we have belonged, at:

- St. Joseph Hospital, Orange, California (Ethics Committee and Perinatal Ethics Committee)
- St. Joseph Healthcare System, Albuquerque, New Mexico
- Harbor-UCLA County Hospital, Torrance, California
- UCLA Medical Center, Los Angeles, California (Ethics Committee and Nursing Ethics Committee)
- Kaiser-Permanente, West Los Angeles, California
- Visiting Nurses Association of Orange County, Orange, California
- St. Jude Medical Center, Fullerton, California
- Queen of the Valley Hospital, Napa, California
- Santa Rosa Memorial Hospital, Santa Rosa, California
- Saint Mary of the Plains, Lubbock, Texas
- Garden Grove Hospital and Medical Center, Garden Grove, California
- Torrance Memorial Medical Center, Torrance, California
- St. Joseph Hospital, Eureka, California
- California Lutheran Homes, Alhambra, California
- Long Beach Veterans Administration Hospital, Long Beach, California
- Humboldt Home Health Ethics Committee, Humboldt, California

1

Taking Stock: Where Ethics Committees Originated and Where They Are Now

It is a puzzling fact that ethics committees are popular in concept and controversial in practice. An understanding of the history, and particularly the origins, of the ethics committee movement might help committee members appreciate this paradox.

The Origins of Ethics Committees

Frequently, ethics committees are criticized as bodies that (1) interfere in or take over decision making regarding patient care and treatment and (2) lack the expertise to do so. Given the ancestry of the committees, these two charges are probably inevitable. In the first published history of the bioethics movement, David Rothman described an ethics committee as one of a group of "strangers" who appeared at patient bedsides in the 1970s and 1980s.[1] The task of these "strangers" was to protect the patient by ensuring that physicians had the patient's best interests in mind when making treatment decisions. According to Rothman, this change in the physician–patient relationship—the addition of a watchdog group—resulted from widely publicized revelations that physician researchers had used patients as their subjects without either the patients' knowledge or their understanding of the risks involved.

In the 1970s, these revelations led to government commissions and to the establishment, by law, of institutional review boards (IRBs), which were charged with reviewing all federally funded research projects to ensure that patients who were research subjects gave genuine informed consent when they agreed to participate in research. This view of the ethics committee as a direct descendant of the IRB is common, in part because both the IRBs and the ethics committees expect some nonphysician representation in their groups and because both are oriented toward the protection of patients. However, it is not the only possible view of how ethics committees came to be.

Ethics committees have at least four potential ancestors in addition to the IRB:

1. *The dialysis patient selection committees* that arose in the 1960s after long-term dialysis became possible but before there was sufficient equipment or reimbursement to cover all patients with end-stage renal disease. These lay committees reviewed patient dossiers and chose from among the medically eligible patients those who were to be given a chance at dialysis. The physicians were then informed as to which patients had been selected.

2. *The prognosis committees* required by the New Jersey Supreme Court in the 1976 *Quinlan* case.[2] In this case, the court held that the hospital should convene an "ethics committee" to determine whether Ms. Quinlan's reported prognosis was correct; that is, to determine whether it was accurate to say, as had been said at trial, that she had no reasonable chance of returning to a cognitive and sapient state. If the committee

concluded that the prognosis was correct, the patient's surrogate was permitted to request that treatment be stopped.

3. *The abortion selection committees* that existed in hospitals in many states prior to the 1973 legalization of abortion in *Roe v. Wade.* These committees were expected to determine whether a pregnant woman who had requested an abortion was likely to risk her life or health if the pregnancy were not terminated. The difficult part of this determination was interpreting what constituted a "threat to health."

4. *The medical–moral committees in Catholic hospitals* that assessed treatment decisions in the light of Catholic teaching. These committees usually dealt with reproductive issues, issues of extraordinary treatment in terminal illness, and the use of analgesics.

No one of these is the true parent of hospital ethics committees while the others are false; all were in the cultural consciousness at the time ethics committees first began to develop in the 1970s. However, this multiple heritage means that ethics committees carry a mixed message about their form, purpose, process, membership, and accountability. Are they to have extensive lay membership (as did the dialysis committees) or minimal lay membership (as do the IRBs)? Is it permissible to have no lay membership (as did the abortion committees)? Is their task to ensure that legal requirements are met (as is the IRB task) or that moral requirements are met (as did the medical–moral committees)? Are they to protect the institution from legal challenge (as the abortion committees were expected to do) or to protect the professionals from making difficult choices (as the dialysis committees and prognosis committees were to do)? Are they to confirm the accuracy of medical judgments (as the prognosis committees did) or to assess the accuracy of the psychosocial judgments behind the treatment decisions (as the abortion committees did)? Because ethics committees have developed spontaneously throughout the country and because ethics committees are similar to but not the same as these ancestors, all these questions can be answered yes, in a sense.

What *can* be said about these ethics committee ancestors is that (1) all were charged with *overseeing decisions* about issues whose resolution involved a considerable degree of conflict in cultural values (or, in the case of the medical–moral committees, the values of a subculture), and (2) four of the five ancestral committees were composed of people chosen for their *specific expertise.* Current ethics committees differ in both respects.

Decision-Making Responsibility

The questions posed to these committees were not easily answered. There was no obvious answer to the question of which patients should be selected for dialysis and which allowed to die; no obvious answer to how to assess the balance between risk to patient and benefit to society in choosing to fund a research project; no obvious answer to how much distress a pregnant woman had to experience or expect before the pregnancy was considered a threat to her health; and no obvious answer to the prickly question of what constituted extraordinary treatment, or when a known and anticipated effect of treatment was intended and when it was only an unintended side (or double) effect.

Only in the case of the *Quinlan*-generated prognosis committee was the answer to the question factual in nature: was Ms. Quinlan likely to return to a cognitive and sapient state? There is some irony in finding that the only ancestor actually called an ethics committee was given no task of ethical analysis. The New Jersey court obtained the idea of an ethics committee from an article by Karen Teel discussing the use of ethics committees to help physicians make difficult treatment decisions for seriously ill newborns.[3] The article incorrectly implied that many such committees existed, and perhaps the court thought it could simply add this prognosis confirmation function to the committee's other activities. The court's secondary purpose for the committee, however, appeared to be to make a hard decision somewhat easier by diffusing responsibility for it among the court, physician, prognosis committee, and patient's family.

In this sense, the prognosis committee joins the other four ethics committee ancestors as groups that were to be responsible for hard decisions by making them, overseeing them, and taking some degree of responsibility for them. These committees are all in some sense a political response to hard questions whose resolution had potential for political (and legal) repercussions. By delegating responsibility to a formally selected group of people, the institutions hoped to prevent hurried, unreflective, or excessively ideological decisions that would harm both patients and institutions and to reassure the public that the decision *was* considered and careful.

This commonality among their ancestry is an important issue (and burden) for current ethics committees, which are, by analogy, perceived as decision makers. However, ethics committees do not have the authority that all five ancestor committees had. For example, the dialysis and abortion committees were authorized by physicians and hospital administrators to select patients for treatment. Institutional review boards were authorized by law to approve only those research protocols that rise to a specific level of information disclosure to obtain informed consent from patient subjects. Medical–moral committees spoke with the authority of the church and the hospital's religious mission, and patients who did not accept those views were free to go to other hospitals.

By contrast, ethics committees have been given no authority by anyone to make any decisions: They are authorized only to discuss treatment decisions and to provide education explaining the ethical standards for such decisions. They may recommend policies and guidelines, but they have no authority to put them into place without the approval of some institutional authority. Yet, the ancestry leaves people with the fear that, in some way, ethics committees will be making decisions and forcing others to accept their views.

The Role of Expertise

Ethics committees are often criticized for not being knowledgeable enough to carry out their mission. Here, too, the origins of ethics committees may create confusion. For example, medical–moral committees were composed of two sets of experts: those who knew the church's teaching and those who knew the medical facts of the cases in which church teaching might be an issue. Abortion committees were usually composed of psychiatrists who were expert in psychological issues and obstetricians who were expert in reproduction. Prognosis committees needed medical expertise to determine prognoses. Internal review boards are dominated by researchers, although there is some requirement for lay participation; in addition, they operate under specific governmental rules.

Only the dialysis committees were composed of nonexperts. As it happens, those committees quickly got into trouble with the public when Shana Alexander wrote about them in *Life* magazine.[4] Subsequent to her article, the committees were accused of taking on God-like powers ("God Committees," the article called them), while using middle-class values to make their decisions. God, by implication, had expertise about how to make such decisions, and mere mortals neither had nor could have such expertise and thus should not be making such decisions.

Ethics committees, arising in the wake of cases such as *Quinlan* and espousing multidisciplinary and nonexpert membership (including nonhospital lawyers, clergy and philosophers, and nonclinical hospital secretaries and maintenance staff members sprinkled among physicians, nurses, social workers, and administrators), are open to the same kind of criticism as the discredited patient selection dialysis committees with respect to expertise (or its absence). The fear of inadequate expertise troubles committee members as well. They worry about whether they know enough and about what it is that they should know more. They are sure they do not know enough ethics, and they doubt that they know enough law.

What is often missing in understanding present ethics committees is that they are not intended to be decision makers or experts in the manner of their ancestor committees. Moreover, the absence of expertise is not a mistake in the creation of ethics committees; indeed, it is an important part of their reason for coming into being.

Ethics Committees as Grass-Roots Phenomena

The ethics committees in hospitals are significantly different from their ancestors in both these aspects, because the impulse that has driven them is largely democratic. That is, it is the belief that a variety of individuals from different backgrounds with different personal and professional perspectives and experiences can come together and openly discuss problematic issues involving conflicting values. Although it was assumed that some decision making would emerge from these discussions, it was also assumed that the actual decision makers would remain the same: the physicians, nurses, patients, and administrators who had come to the committee were expected to leave with the same responsibilities they had brought with them. The process of discussion was expected to change their understanding in some way. For example, discussion might lead them to consider a different course of action than they had originally proposed, or it might cause them to have greater confidence in the course of action they had originally intended to pursue. However, the point of the committee discussion was and is *process* not *product, forum* not *decision.*

This is the principal element that distinguishes ethics committees from their ancestors. This is why "multidisciplinarity" has been such an important factor in their formation. And this is why the movement has been content with having ethics committee members who do not have degrees or certification in bioethics. Members may find such educational pursuits interesting and rewarding, but they should not be necessary. Just as ethics committees are not about decision making (but are about the process of thinking about decisions), they are not about expertise (but are about the process of sharing knowledge). In a sense, they are antiexpertise: That is their democratic nature.

Yet, in a world in which decision making and expertise are highly valued and rewarded (as they are in contemporary American culture and in health care institutions in particular), the temptation of ethics committees to be perceived by both others and themselves as ethical decision-making experts is always there. Their ancestry and the institutional context make this temptation doubly difficult to resist. However, the long-term strength of ethics committees is in their grass-roots nature and their democratic makeup, in the breadth of their knowledge, and in their understanding of their own community—not in their claim to health care ethics decision-making expertise.

Salient Features of Current Ethics Committees

Where are ethics committees in the 1990s? Speakers and writers often talk about ethics committees as if they were a single phenomenon, uniform throughout the country, which leaves the impression that a great deal is known about them. What is known is that most are involved in education, policy and guideline recommendation, and some case review.

Beyond that, however, virtually no data exist about the real-life functioning of the more than 4,000 institutional ethics committees in the United States. Most of the existing information is anecdotal, from individual committee members. Many ethics committees are isolated from one another, and their members are largely unaware of any ties to a larger movement of ethics committees and even of bioethics. However, even if there were data available, the fact that some ethics committees are newly created, others a few years old, and still others well into their second decade would make those data difficult to understand, as it is likely that committee experiences differ markedly.

In a recent survey of approximately 20 medical ethics committees nationwide, Gibson found both similarities and differences among them.[5] These committees represented hospitals ranging in size from 130 to 650 beds. The committees themselves had between 10 and 25 members. Most committees shared basic values. They described themselves as interdisciplinary both in makeup and approach. They wished to avoid appearing intrusive in case consultations, and they believed that the parties (usually patients, families, and health care professionals) rather than the committee itself should make the final decision in case consultations. Most also viewed ongoing education as a major, if not the primary, function of the committee in the health care institution.

Despite the common issues, the committees surveyed exhibited broad differences in their views of their institutional roles, their roles in case consultation, and in the ways they functioned. For example, some described themselves as "exclusive" in membership, limiting membership to only a few professions; others described themselves as "inclusive," attempting to involve as many representatives of the hospital and even the wider community as possible. Those committees viewing their roles as primarily educational tended to be composed of persons with a wide variety of substantive expertise, whereas those seeing their roles as helping with specific (mostly patient care) problems in the institution tended to be composed largely of institutional and professional (physician) representatives.

Probably because ethics committees are so isolated, members are very interested in knowing what is happening in other committees—whether their experiences are typical or different from those of others. Eventually, research will be able to provide more of this information, but in its absence, we offer our collective impressions of ethics committees at this time, acknowledging (and cautioning the reader about) the limitation of generalizations.

Committee Membership

In general, although ethics committees "look" multidisciplinary, nurses tend to be underrepresented. We use the term *underrepresented* in two senses: statistically underrepresented, considering that there are many more nurses in health care than in any other profession; and underrepresented in terms of the frequency with which nurses report confronting ethical dilemmas or problems. Many committees with 15 or so members have only one or two nurses. Some committees have successfully involved clergy from outside the hospital's chaplaincy or pastoral care office; many have not. Lay members are not the rule on committees. However, if the committee has a lay member, this individual is often very sophisticated with respect to the issues (for example, a gerontologist, an ethics teacher, a hospice director in a program not related to the institution in question, and so on). Generally, lay members are considered to be persons not employed by the institution, but not necessarily persons who represent the views of the community in which the institution is located.

Committee Functions

Some committees have chosen to do no case review and others are not involved in policy writing; but most committees divide their time among the three functions—education, case review, and policy and guideline recommendation. However, education is more likely to be self-education, policy writing (other than forgoing treatment) is likely to be at the request of others in the institution, and case review is likely to be sporadic.

Education

Some older committees have managed to institute regular educational programs (for example, monthly forums or grand rounds in the institution) or once-a-year extended programs during bioethics week. A few committees have experimented with regular publication of articles on bioethics and the committee in either the hospital's newsletter or an ethics committee newsletter. Occasional grand rounds are not uncommon. However, most committees focus on self-education. Fewer committees have been involved in education around the Patient Self-Determination Act than might be expected. This may be because education under this act was perceived as a *legal* issue rather than an *ethical* one, and thus was turned over to the administration.

Policy and Guideline Recommendation

Do-not-resuscitate (DNR) policies continue to be the bread and butter of policy writing, with recent emphasis on DNR in surgery, DNR in the event of iatrogenic cardiopulmonary arrest, futile cardiopulmonary resuscitation (CPR), and the status of DNR orders for patients who are transferred from one facility to another or from home to the institution. Because policies on forgoing treatment and advance directives are required under the federal Patient Self-Determination Act, most committees that have not previously written such policies are now undertaking them. Policies addressing treatment of seriously ill newborns are common in hospitals with tertiary care nurseries. Policies dealing with the "demanding patient" (or more often the demanding family member, for example, a situation in which the patient and/or family wants a specific form of treatment that physicians believe is not indicated) are rare. A few committees are trying to determine whether they can help to address these issues in a professional rather than an economic context. That is, they are writing policies that may restrict patient access to treatment not because it is expensive but because it is not medically appropriate in terms of the goals of medicine as a profession. Treatment of rape victims, forgoing of nutrition and hydration, pain control for the terminally ill patient, confidentiality of and access to medical records, and (to a lesser extent) policies involving HIV testing are other issues in which ethics committees are involved.

Issues of pain control for patients with chronic (as opposed to acute) pain are beginning to be addressed, with concerns about the meaning of addiction in such patients moving to the forefront. A few committees have taken on problems involved with surrogacy (who consents to treatment and even who takes the child home). Issues involving ethics in psychiatric practice are still infrequently addressed, even in institutions that have mental health units. Few committees are involved with ethical questions concerning consent and confidentiality in the treatment of adolescents.

Where there is a reasonably broad social consensus on a specific topic, policy writing is a task that ethics committees handle quite easily. Where no such consensus has yet developed, the committees move much more slowly. This may result from fear of legal consequences or from uncertainty about the committees' authority to take a stand on an issue where consensus has not yet been reached. When committees do become involved in such unresolved areas, they usually cast a broad consultative net so that they do not move in advance of their hospital community.

Case Review/Consultation

Older committees, particularly those that have had negative experiences with case review involving the entire committee, are beginning to create core consultation teams to handle consultations. Most committees would like to do more consultation and, although someone always says that it would be impossible to call a meeting on short notice, when such a meeting is called, the turnout is usually excellent. Physicians in some hospitals are beginning to write orders to "request ethics committee consult," a development that may be problematic for ethics committees in that the request may be less for a discussion forum than for something along the lines of a medical consultation.

Institutional Support

Most committees have administrative support in the form of secretarial assistance in keeping minutes, doing copying, and mailing out agendas and meeting notices; and financial assistance in providing some educational materials (books, journal subscriptions, and so on), food for committee meetings (sometimes only coffee and cookies, sometimes full meals), and parking, if necessary, for off-site members. A few committees have their own small budgets and thus must decide how much duplication of written materials is really necessary, and what books and publications their members will actually read if the committee buys them. Without this minimal level of support, the committee is not likely to function very well or for very long. It should be noted that ethics committees in their early incarnation as study groups rarely received this kind of support. However, if the group is to turn into a functioning hospital ethics committee, tangible economic support is vital.

If the administration or medical staff committee wishes to see the ethics committee flourish rather than just exist, there must be additional resources; for example, full or partial tuition fees for ethics committee or ethics-related conferences and workshops, outside consultants for evaluating the committee or educating the committee in particular areas, and an ethics resource person — either an individual at the corporate level who serves a number of hospitals, an individual who serves a number of geographically close but legally unrelated institutions, or an individual within the institution who has obtained special training in the field and whose job description includes the charge to devote some specific portion of his or her time solely to ethics. A committee that does not have reasonable access to an ethics resource person may become too isolated from the larger world of health care ethics to be able to ensure its growth and development. If this committee does not die, it will at least wither.

Committee Morale

Some ethics committees are experiencing loss of morale. The *Medical Ethics Advisor* suggests that this results from loss of initial enthusiasm, realization of the problems committees face, case consultations with the same problem again and again, absence of group cohesiveness, failure to act aggressively, impatience, and being outside the mainstream of the field.[6] This may also be a time in which there is a shakeout of members, with those who have a sustained interest in these issues remaining on the committee and those with a different kind or level of interest leaving. It is certainly the case that older committees often do not have the same kind of enthusiasm or liveliness that they had five or six years ago; but it is also true that at least some of those committees have developed into effective working groups that meet more frequently and get more done, even if it is in a quieter way.

Morale is related to expectations, and in a new area such as this, many people are likely to have expectations that do not work out. It does not prove that ethics committees do not work or are a bad idea; it only proves that expectations did not match up with reality. Committees can then move to change either the expectations or the reality. The authors hope that this book will contribute to both kinds of change.

Nursing Ethics Committees

Ethics committees for nurses only are becoming more common in acute care hospitals. These committees deal exclusively with ethical issues from a nursing perspective. They are primarily educational in nature but may also do retrospective case review, both as an educational effort to help nurses understand these issues in light of various value conflicts and to help nurses consider how to act in the future so that they can more effectively deal with ethical conflicts.

Nursing is perceived as a field in which at least some of the burnout results from insufficient authority to address ethical conflicts, and nursing ethics committees try to help nurses use the resources they have to reduce feelings of powerlessness. When nursing ethics committees are asked to discuss a case that needs to be addressed more broadly, they are free to (and even expected to) bring this case to the attention of the hospital ethics committee with its broader membership base and its clearer role in hospital administrative or medical staff structures.

Nurses who have been involved in nursing ethics committees are generally very enthusiastic about their experiences, and do not perceive themselves as being in an antagonistic relationship to hospital ethics committees already functioning in their institutions. Usually the chairs of the nursing ethics committee are also members of the hospital ethics committee and perceive one of their roles on that committee to be the conveyer of information to their larger nursing constituency.

Community Agency Ethics Committees

Occasionally ethics committees have been established in some home health care programs, in hospice programs, and in community agencies, but they function differently because their institutional structure differs considerably from that of acute care hospitals. Physicians are much less likely to participate, let alone dominate, such committees. Nursing and other staff are often mobile and patients are usually not in a single facility, so there is less common knowledge about the patients. These community agencies tend to be more heavily involved in both the patient's medical care and the patient's and family's life than are committees in acute care facilities, and ethical issues tend to spill over into much broader areas.

Greater exposure to families tends to make family involvement in decision making for the patient more problematic. For example, as staff become more aware of the nature and extent of family dysfunction that sometimes exists in the face of serious illness, turning to the family for decisions becomes a much more uncertain matter. Issues of assisted suicide appear to be more common and more subtle than in the acute care setting because questions of responsibility are less clear when the patient is, for example, at home rather than in the professional's facility. A sensitivity to community ethics (for example, of the family as community) rather than to individualistic ethics may understandably underlie the ethos of such agencies, but may be at odds with the general thrust of bioethics, which is so strongly oriented to the individual alone.

Ethics Committees in Long-Term Care Facilities

The fastest growth in ethics committees is expected to occur in extended care over the next five years. These ethics committees have often been helped into existence by acute care hospital committees, but, apart from their shared concern with forgoing treatment issues, long-term care committees will probably develop along different lines.

The differences between these institutions are considerable: physicians are likely to play a minor role (although they need to be included at some level in the ethics committee) and administrators are likely to be much more dominant. Levels of staff education generally will be lower, and there may well be greater cultural and class differences between staff and patients and their families than in the acute care setting. Frequently, long-term care facilities are so heavily regulated that their concerns (if not their needs) are more directly focused on legal rather than ethical issues: it is not helpful to patients if the facility is always in trouble with the state. In addition, they are often part of multistate corporations whose policies are issued from a central legal headquarters. Often, there is a bias toward very conservative approaches to all questions, making it difficult for individual long-term care facilities to exercise their own solutions to ethical issues in patient care as they see them in their own setting. Long-term care ethics committees deal with medical ethics issues, but are much more likely to have to consider issues of daily life (for example, roommate assignments, use of telephones, resident access to possessions, and so on).

Ethics Committee Networks

Networks of ethics committees have begun to arise throughout the country. In the spring of 1989, a national meeting of individuals involved in various networks was held in Chicago under the sponsorship of a grant from the Fund for the Improvement of Post-Secondary Education (FIPSE). Networks from Vermont, New Mexico, Arizona, Wisconsin, the San Francisco Bay area, Orange County (CA), Los Angeles County, the Midwest, Minnesota, the Delaware Valley, Washington–Oregon, Connecticut, Michigan, and the U.S. Veterans Administration Hospitals were represented at this meeting. These networks were in various stages of development, and since that time other areas (for example, New York, Maryland, and North Dakota) have reported the establishment of new networks. Networks are usually located in, and in some way supported by, university medical centers or hospital system ethics centers. However, at least one is allied with a state medical association, another with a hospital trade organization, and a third with a freestanding ethics center.

The networks have a variety of activities. Some conduct educational programs (ranging from occasional to regular and intensive programs) for their constituents, some produce regular publications, some carry out surveys, some provide a community forum for discussing the successes and problems of individual ethics committees, and some have ventured into communitywide solutions to problems that are experienced by all institutions (for example, recognition of DNR orders by paramedics in the community). Michigan's network provides nationwide access to an electronic bulletin board.

However, the focus of all networks is to develop some sense of larger community relationships among institutional ethics committees (whether in acute care hospitals, long-term care facilities, or intrainstitutional groups). Some involve membership fees or program fees; others operate without any specific income, depending on individuals volunteering time on behalf of their employing agencies. For the most part, their structures appear to be fairly informal. There are few written reports of the networks other than in their own publications. *HEC [HealthCare Ethics Committee] Forum* has published several reports from networks,[7] and in 1992 began a regular section on Ethics Committee Network News.

Conclusion

Apart from the differences arising from variations in the nature of institutions, there are great differences among ethics committees at every level with respect to the perceived legitimacy of the committee and its work, the visibility of the committee, the scope of its responsibility, the clarity of its mission, the commitment of its members, and even its size. There are successful committees with 10 members and successful committees with 40 and more members. Some committees have had virtually the same members from their beginning; others rotate members like clockwork. Some meet at 7:00 in the morning, some at noontime, others over dinner. Some do no consultation; some no policy writing. Some are asked to become involved in institutional issues that were not thought to be part of the ethics committee mandate (ethics of new business plans, for example). Some are virtually unknown to the hospital administration. Some committees interview prospective participants in in vitro fertilization and surrogacy programs to ensure that patients are giving genuine informed consent. Others write policies advising the hospital not to honor surrogacy contracts but to look to the woman who gave birth for all decisions. Many committees are actively involved in educating their communities about advance directives and the Patient Self-Determination Act, and many are not.

What is most impressive about committees at this time is their range of responses to the charges they have been given. The grass-roots nature of ethics committees means that there is great opportunity for individual initiative and creativity as well as for selectivity in determining what is important and achievable in a specific institution. Committees should use this freedom to shape their mission to their institution, to document their work in order to legitimize it, and to reach out to others engaged in similar work in order to share their knowledge and experience.

Exercises

Use the following questions as a starting point for a focused discussion in your committee.

1. How much concern is there among members that the committee's work not only serve to protect the patient's interests but also clearly *appear* to protect the patient's interests. That is, is the committee particularly concerned that there be no appearance of serving the institution's interest (particularly its financial interests)? What kinds of cases or policies would create such conflict?
2. Should the committee be asked by the administration to take on tasks that seem to be less patient centered than institution centered? Is the committee's sole function to protect patient interests?
3. Is there resistance to having an ethics committee in your institution? What is the source of that resistance? What can be done to overcome it?
4. Is there a sense in the institution that ethics committees do not have any special kind of knowledge because everyone in the institution is ethical?
5. Do physicians and nurses in your institution generally have close and cooperative working relationships that make it easier to break down the hierarchical chain of command in the committee itself?

6. Does the committee have a distinctly group feel (for example, members are comfortable with one another and sense a common mission) but still exist in some isolation from the rest of the institution?
7. Is the committee generally encouraged by the administration or the medical executive committee but given little guidance and few or no resources to support its work?
8. Is the committee well known in the institution? Does that matter?

Notes and References

1. Rothman, D. *Strangers at the Bedside*. New York City: Basic Books, 1991.

2. *In the matter of Karen Quinlan,* 70 NJ 10, 1976.

3. Teel, K. The physician's dilemma. A doctor's view: what the law should be. *Baylor Law Review* 27:6, 1975.

4. They decide who lives, who dies. *Life,* Nov. 9, 1962, p. 102.

5. Gibson, J. M. Unpublished survey, Albuquerque, University of New Mexico, 1989–1990.

6. Is your committee losing the enthusiasm it once had? *Medical Ethics Advisor* 7(5):57ff., May 1991.

7. See, for example, Iserson, K. Strategic planning for bioethics committees and networks. *HEC Forum* 3(3):117–28, 1991; and Miller, R. B., Gawron, T. W., Pitts, R. T., Bade R. H., O'Rourke, B., Rasinski-Gregory, D. C., and Aleman, M. Development of a county pre-hospital DNR program: contributions of a bioethics network. *HEC Forum* 4(3):175–86, 1992. See also *Hastings Center Report* 20(2):33–34, 1990.

2

The Role of Ethics Committees: Going beyond Life-Sustaining Treatment

It is one thing to say that ethics committees should conduct education on ethical issues, recommend policies that are ethically important, and review cases with respect to ethical issues. It is another thing to determine exactly what activities can fulfill that mission. New committees tend to restrict themselves to self-education; after completing that phase, they devote time to educating others, to hearing cases (often only retrospectively), and to writing policies that are requested. More mature committees tend to broaden their notion of the issues identified as "ethical." They may consider pain management, nurse–physician communication, or patient education in areas other than forgoing treatment. They also tend to be more personally aware of, and responsive to, issues as opposed to waiting for an issue or a concern to be brought to them.

A Shift in Perspective

A committee that has worked on self-education for a while may be familiar with the basic ethical principles related to the physician–patient or nurse–patient relationship. But it may be less confident about viewing ethical issues in a more comprehensive manner. For example, committee members may be fairly confident about dealing with a particular issue at the individual level, but much less confident about dealing with the same issue on an institutional or societal level. Thus, members need to become adept at shifting their ethical perspective. Some issues are better addressed at the individual level, others at the institutional level, and still others at the societal level. For example, in a case where a patient or family is receiving different or inconsistent information from various caregivers, it may be necessary to address the problem at the individual level. However, if the problem stems from the way nurses and physicians relate to one another and to patients in this institution (rather than from the dynamics of this particular patient/family/caregiver), this problem would be better addressed at the institutional level. Committee members might question whether a particular problem with which they are dealing results primarily from the behavior of individuals or from organizational structures and systems. The answer to that question should affect how the committee thinks about the problem and how it chooses to address it.

Identification of Institutional Issues

Once the committee is confident in its ability to sort out individual, institutional, and societal problems, it is ready to take the next step. That is, the committee needs to improve its ability to identify ethical issues that are less obvious and often ignored but that have a profound impact on people's experiences in the institution. Committees that are beginning to move away from a more literal view of ethics might want to reflect on such questions as:

- What is it like to be a patient or family in this institution?
- What is it like to be employed by this institution?
- What is it like to teach at or be taught in this institution?
- What is it like to practice medicine or nursing in this institution?
- To what extent does this institution seek to humanize these experiences?

Committees might also want to look at the following:

- Where and how people wait for care
- Where and how families are given bad news and asked to make decisions
- Privacy of information and person
- The language we use when speaking about patients, especially those who are very sick, old, or demented
- The way we respond to patients of different ethnic backgrounds, including our efforts to achieve good communication
- Status symbols among/between staff members

If every committee member made it a point to observe these and other similar issues, to reflect on them, and to report their perceptions at each meeting, the committee would have far more impact than an occasional case review. The experience would heighten members' awareness of what it means to speak of the institution as an ethical community. A significant criticism leveled at ethics committees has been that the institution's ethics may be seen to reside exclusively in the ethics committee. A parallel problem for ethics committee members is that ethical issues may be seen to reside only in policy and case review.

Although the ethics committee's mission may not be to resolve all ethical issues in the institution, it should encompass an awareness of such issues. For example, the ethics committee may not be able to require that the institution's infertility program have a clear protocol for deciding who is and who is not eligible for its services and that this protocol be ethically justified; however, the committee should know whether such a protocol exists and should understand the ethical ramifications of not having one. If a protocol does not exist, the committee may want to exercise one of several options: to issue a brief paper explaining its concerns to the program staff, to use the issue as a basis for a general educational effort in the institution, or simply to ensure that its members are fully versed on the general issue. The action taken by the committee must relate to its own particular situation.

Members sometimes feel that their committee has gotten stuck in end-of-life treatment decisions and that this is the only issue they are supposed to be concerned about. "We need to know more," said one family practice physician. "We need to talk about truth telling, about confidentiality, . . . about what you're supposed to do when your patient tells you that he is gay but asks you not to put it in his chart."

The problems with such issues seem to be that there is either little discussion of them in the literature or very little consensus about them in the field. It is as if ethics committees are saying, "Well, if the *experts* don't know the answer, what are we supposed to be doing?" But this attitude about "expertise" needs to be guarded against. Ethics committees are multidisciplinary just because it was thought that, when an issue arose that was unfamiliar or for which there was no standard response, the voices of many from different perspectives would help the group arrive at some consensus that seemed ethically acceptable. It is only over time that what now seem to be easy issues (for example, most DNR decisions) became easy. The most difficult part is beginning where no one knows quite what to think, where no one has enough facts or even knows what facts he or she needs. It is there, however, that the mature ethics committee can make a contribution and expand its institution's understanding of ethics in health care.

Suggested Activities

The following are suggestions for activities that an ethics committee might undertake. The list is not exclusive. Some are activities that ethics committees have already done; others are activities that they could do. Each committee can use this list as a starting point for developing its own agenda:

- Hold regularly scheduled (monthly or quarterly) educational meetings for the hospital community. These meetings could involve a case discussion, a videotape, a presentation of a policy developed by the ethics committee, a discussion of an ethical issue currently in the news media, and so on.
- Conduct a written survey of hospital staff to assess awareness, interests, attitudes, or perceived problems in the area of bioethics.
- Establish annual goals for the ethics committee and periodically assess whether progress is being made toward achieving them.
- Establish an annual calendar and assign a different member of the ethics committee each month or at various times during the year to discuss an article, a case study, and so on—either of the member's choice or one assigned. This would spread responsibility for education, ensure that at least a portion of the agenda will be educational, and assist members to become aware of and knowledgeable about ethical issues as they prepare for their month's responsibilities.
- Have each member of the committee organize a meeting in his or her respective department on an ethical issue of concern to the members of that department.
- Perform an audit of policies that have been recommended by the committee. Are they being followed? Do people know about them? Are the required patient chart notes being made?
- Develop a brochure for patients and families about how treatment decisions are made, about advance directives, and/or about the ethics committee's role in the hospital.
- Develop an effective half-hour educational program and offer to take it around to departments or nursing units throughout the hospital.
- Arrange meetings with nursing department managers or head nurses to discuss ethical issues that arise in the various units. Explore ways the ethics committee might help nurse managers to develop their own skills in resolving some of these issues.
- Conduct an ethics study group for nurses only.
- Conduct an ethics study group for physicians only.
- Initiate a literature and health care discussion group for interested physicians and staff.
- Invite ethics committee members from other area institutions to attend a session to discuss mutual goals, problems, and concerns. This could lead to the formation of an ethics committee network.
- Invite members of another local ethics committee to make a presentation to describe their committee's activities.
- Invite members of another local ethics committee to help evaluate the institution's ethics committee meetings. (They can act as knowledgeable but sympathetic outsiders.)
- Offer to provide speakers for local clubs and service organizations. Topics might include helping the community to understand ethical issues or the role of ethics committees in area hospitals.
- Conduct a self-evaluation in which individual members evaluate their own contributions to the ethics committee and reflect on their hopes for its future.
- Develop a formal orientation program for all new ethics committee members.
- Join together with ethics committees from several nearby institutions to develop and conduct a formal orientation program for all new ethics committee members.
- Contact nursing homes in the area to which patients are likely to be transferred and develop communication regarding patient/family wishes about treatment when patients are transferred between facilities.
- Offer to help a long-term care institution in the development of its ethics committee.

- Have each committee member reflect on what he or she thinks are the five or six most important ethical issues or situations in the institution. Share these with all members at a meeting and decide which, if any, of these issues the ethics committee should become involved with and which ones they should refer to someone else.
- Think about whether there are policies or guidelines that the committee has not developed but should be developing.
- Develop a short summary of all the hospital policies that have significant ethical content. Make the summary available to physicians and staff.
- Write a regular column for the hospital newsletter informing the community about new policies, new court cases, and controversial topics in bioethics and what the hospital is doing or might do about them.
- Distribute an occasional information sheet to hospital staff and physicians updating them on important committee work or ethical issues.
- Stock and regularly update a centrally located bulletin board with articles and announcements regarding ethics and health care.
- Summarize important articles in the ethics literature for distribution to selected staff and physicians.
- Hold a bioethics week with a special activity each day. Be sure to include activities for those on the night shift as well.
- Study body language and its meaning for communication.
- Take a course in mediation or other kinds of conflict resolution.
- Invite social scientists or behavioral psychologists to address the committee on how to develop a better understanding of conflict resolution, communication styles, group dynamics, or effective public speaking to enhance education efforts.
- Invite a sociologist to work with the committee to develop a sociogram of the group in order to elucidate the various relationships within the committee that affect its work.
- Discuss Meyers–Briggs tests to help understand various styles of conflict resolution.
- Investigate the user-friendliness of the institution for non–English speakers and for individuals with disabilities, including the hearing impaired, the blind, and those confined to wheelchairs.
- Sponsor a day in which staff "take on" disabilities for a period of time in order to help them better understand the problems of their patients with disabilities.
- Write a song about bioethics.
- Assess the institution's decor from the patient's perspective.
- Have an intensivist provide a hands-on demonstration of what being an ICU patient involves. The demonstration should include discussion of what is routinely done and why.
- Have committee members read a chapter of *Bed Number Ten* by Baier and Schomaker[1] and discuss what it is like to be an ICU patient from the patient's perspective.
- Interview patients and families about the transfer of patients from various units to an ICU. What is this experience like for patients and families?
- Survey patients and families about their experiences in the hospital.
- Request copies of letters (with names removed) written to the hospital or to the patient representative office to learn what patients and families find troubling or especially rewarding about their hospital experiences.
- Visit a nursing home to find out how it operates.
- Visit a hospice program and a home health agency to find out how they work.
- Invite a nursing home, hospice, or home health care staff member to speak to the ethics committee on the ethical problems that arise in those settings.
- Ask patients or families who earlier consulted the committee about treatment decisions to come back at a later date to discuss how the experience could have been more helpful.
- Invite physicians, nurses, and/or other health care team members who have been patients in the institution to talk to the committee about their experiences as patients.

- Have the ethics committee and a community agency jointly sponsor a forum, a day-long event, or a week-long series of events to increase understanding of ethical issues in health care.
- Hold weekly brown-bag lunches in an informal setting and discuss landmark cases.
- Arrange programs for area clergy to help them understand the ethical aspects of treatment decisions in the hospital setting. Consider doing this in cooperation with the hospital chaplaincy service.
- Work with area clergy to help them understand the need for and the role of advance directives.
- Hold an open forum (one ethics committee calls these forums "ethics hearings") in which people can talk about their concerns about ethical issues in patient care.
- Ask to be put on the agenda of other hospital committees so that an ethics committee member not only can explain what the committee is and what it does, but also discuss how its work might be coordinated with the work of other hospital committees.
- Decide as a matter of policy to call everyone on the committee by his or her first name. Discuss what this means. Consider how this affects the use of names outside the committee.
- Make a list of all the kinds of power and authority in the hospital (starting with degrees/education level, expertise, gender, seniority, title, control of resources, and so on). Have members candidly assess themselves as to how many of these powers they have. Discuss the kinds of power and authority that patients and families have in the hospital or on the committee.
- Consider whether the role of the ethics committee is to work as an "expert on call" or as a force for change in the institution. Which does the committee itself want its role to be? What does the administration or medical staff want the committee to be? Are there other options?
- If the committee is interested in being a force for change, seek out specialists in organizational development to help committee members better understand this objective.
- If the committee is interested in being an expert on-call consultant, seek out those who can explain how specialized consultation works. Some useful books include *Ethics at the Bedside*[2] and *Ethics Consultation in Health Care.*[3]
- Organize a panel of knowledgeable individuals, including a hospice nurse, to educate the committee about pain relief. For example, how are issues of chronic pain control handled in the hospital? What are the ethical issues involved in effective pain control? Are they different depending on whether the pain is acute (in terminal care) or chronic?
- Develop a protocol for ensuring that terminally ill patients are adequately treated for acute pain.
- Determine who is responsible for various levels of ethical reality in the institution. Find out what ethical issues the board of trustees regularly addresses and with what ethical issues senior management deals. How does the committee's work relate to that of the board and management with respect to ethical issues? Do members of the ethics committee see themselves as a disconnected island or as a part of the main body of land?
- Have a nurse, physician, and/or social worker demonstrate for the committee how he or she talks with patients about advance directives, explains terminal care decisions, or delivers bad news. Ask members of the committee to role-play the patients.
- Develop brochures on forgoing treatment decisions, advance directives, CPR and DNR orders, case consultation, or other relevant topics for patients. Test them for readability with patients and family members before printing them.
- Find out whether patients and families know about the hospital's ethics committee. If they do not, ask them what they would want from a hospital ethics committee.
- Invite members of other ethics committees to meet on a regular basis to share information.
- Request that each department head come to a meeting to advise the committee on the ethical issues that are important in his or her department.

- Help nurses develop a nursing ethics forum.
- Ask a local legislator to explain the state's interest in ethical issues in health care.
- Find out how house staff and medical students view the patients' hospital experience. Is their idea of what it is like to be a patient different from that of the regular staff or attending or private physicians?
- Survey committee members regularly on some aspect of the ethics committee's work. Get the results back to them in a timely fashion.
- Sponsor a meeting of the ethics committee, hospital chaplains, and area clergy to discuss one another's needs, perspectives, and potential for cooperative action.
- *Think* about. . . .
- *Ask* about. . . .
- *Find out* about. . . .

This list could go on for many pages in increasing detail discussing whom to talk to, what to read, and what to do. Most committees are boxed in by the listing of functions—the education, policy-writing, case-consulting mantra. What makes an ethics committee an exciting and interesting group to belong to is the sense that what members are doing is important to people. Each committee must find out what is of most interest and importance to it, as well as what is available to its members in terms of time, skills, expert personnel, financial resources, and administrative discretion. It is from this diversity that ethics committees will flourish.

Conclusion

What is always apparent when ethics committee members are surveyed is how much their membership means to them. They care about whether the committee succeeds or fails, which is not the case with many other committees. Moreover, the members care about contributing to the committee's success. There is so much goodwill out there, but without taking hold of some kind of project, goodwill cannot be translated into an effective committee—an ethics committee on the move instead of one simply struggling through the mire of uncertainty about its role. When a committee cares about doing consultation, it develops good skills, goodwill, and good protocols. It then thinks about finding ways to help those who have ethics questions reach the committee. When consultation is not what hospital colleagues need from the ethics committee, members should seek out another activity that will help them learn more about what it means to practice in a profession that has a primary commitment to altruism and an ongoing concern for helping others. That is why most health care professionals went into the field in the first place. The ethics committee can help itself and its colleagues keep that ideal alive.

References

1. Baier, S., and Schomaker, M. Z. *Bed Number Ten*. Boca Raton, FL: Corporate Press, 1986.

2. Culver, C. M., editor. *Ethics at the Bedside*. Hanover, NH: University Press of New England, 1990.

3. Fletcher, J., Quist, N., and Jonsen, A., editors. *Ethics Consultation in Health Care*. Ann Arbor, MI: Health Administration Press, 1989.

3

Ethics for Committees: Understanding Ethics and Methodology

Working in an interdisciplinary field means that one must know something about several fields. In bioethics, one must, at a minimum, know something about medicine, nursing, health law, health care financing, societal resources for health care professionals and patients, cultural and religious values, and ethics or ethical analysis. Because members of ethics committees are "working in bioethics," they need to learn about these areas in order to be effective.

It seems obvious to say that ethics committee members need to know about ethics. Yet, it is the most problematic area. One of the most common complaints heard from new (and not so new) ethics committee members after they have returned from attending conferences and workshops is "I wish they had focused more on ethics." Ethics committee members almost never feel they know enough about ethics in general, although they may feel comfortable about the ethics of a particular issue (such as forgoing treatment) on which there is widespread consensus.

It may be that ethics committee members believe they do not know enough about ethics because they misunderstand the nature of both ethics and ethical analysis. Ethical practice, like medical practice and nursing practice, may ultimately be more of an art than a science, which does not mean that it is all just a matter of opinion. Like medical practice and nursing practice, ethical practice requires an understanding of a variety of rules, principles, relationships, and actions and consequences.

The widespread use of Beauchamp's and Childress's *The Principles of Bioethics*[1] (now in its third edition) has created the illusion that if only one could master the principles and some unspecified accompanying method of analysis, the solutions to difficult treatment decisions would be more obvious. In fact, formal ethical analysis and the principles of ethics have been far less helpful to bioethics than many originally expected. Nevertheless, many ethics committee members continue to think that there is a body of knowledge about ethics out there, and if they could only latch onto it, everything would fall into place. They hope for something that does not exist—a relatively clear set of rules that, if followed, produces answers. There are principles and rules and ways of analyzing arguments, but there is no single simple methodology of ethical analysis that does the trick.

The ethical consensus regarding forgoing life-sustaining treatment was developed largely on the principled claim that patient autonomy was more important than the professionals' duty to do no harm (nonmaleficence). This claim was supported by the argument that treatment forgone at the patient's request also served the patient's best interests (thus honoring the duty of beneficence) because the patient is the best judge of those interests. This consensus—developed through the literature, public commissions, and public meetings, and sanctioned by court opinions—suggested that ethical analysis using the principles of patient autonomy, professional beneficence, and justice would be an adequate method for resolving differences. However, these principles have not brought a similar consensus in many other areas, including treatment of seriously ill newborns, appropriate use of new reproductive technologies, conflicts between health care teams and family surrogates with respect to what is in patients' best interests, HIV testing for health care professionals, decisions about futile treatment, as well as many other situations in which the presenting issue is more complex than a disagreement between a physician and a competent patient about continued treatment. Thus, reliance on the principles of bioethics has not brought forth clear consensus.

The inadequacy of looking to either rules and principles or consequences (the second major method of ethical analysis) to determine "right" action in specific situations has led many in bioethics to advocate other approaches to ethical analysis. Ethics committee members may hear references to feminist ethics, ethics of caring, clinical ethics, narrative ethics, casuistry, and virtue ethics, to name only a few of the current favorites. Those who propose these theories offer a richer set of ideas to approach health care decision making, but also create a more frustrating task. If an ethics committee is to "do ethics," how is it to choose from among these methods?

Good ethics committee work is nourished by an understanding of the theory and method discussed in the bioethics literature, but is not driven by it. That is, deliberations and discussions are more thoughtful and more thorough when members know something about these different views of ethical analysis than when they try to use only the principles of bioethics or to force every situation into a procrustean bed of patient autonomy. Knowing about feminist ethics and its emphasis on preserving relationships when resolving conflicts, for example, helps members not only to bring forward their knowledge about relationships in a family and to assess how various options may affect those relationships, but also to value that knowledge as an important part of the ethical dimensions of health care.

Ethics committee work should be informed by this broader understanding of ethical analysis. In addition, it must be guided by good fact-finding, good communication, good judgment, good listening and facilitation skills, an appreciation of the importance of others' perceptions and understandings, and an appropriate level of humility. Ethical theory and method is but one part of this larger set of skills and attitudes, and ethics committees' use of theory and method does not require them to be philosophers, nor does it turn them into ethics experts.

If the ethics committee is doing its job well, it will be seen not as a group of "ethics experts" but rather as a community where issues concerning human dignity and respect can be safely discussed, and where those responsible for patient care decisions can formulate solutions. The committee can model what it hopes for the rest of the hospital: respectful interdisciplinary dialogue, identification of problems and their sources, exploration of options and alternatives for resolution, and the creation of a climate in which conflict and disagreement can be seen as an opportunity for growth rather than as something to be avoided or an opportunity to reinforce status differences. The discussions will focus on reasons for making one choice rather than another. For example: Are the reasons good ones? Can they be defended? Are they consistent with other arguments that could be made? Regardless of theory, ethical analysis depends on articulating and defending reasons for choices.

Realms of Ethical Analysis

Before discussing some of the more prominent theories of ethical analysis, a few words should be said about the *realms* of ethical analysis. Ethical problems can occur at the individual, institutional, or societal level. For example, deciding whether a particular patient should be recommended for a heart transplant is a problem of individual ethics; deciding whether an institution should limit the categories of patients whom it will consider for heart transplantation (for example, only those who can pay) is a problem of institutional ethics; and deciding whether private or public health insurance coverage should include heart transplantation is a problem of societal ethics.

Ethics committees were created (if only implicitly) to address ethical issues in the care of individual patients. More recently, they have been asked or have chosen to address problems at the institutional level (for example, whether the institution should restrict access to a very expensive drug on the basis of the patient's expected quality of life) and at the societal level (for example, whether the ethics committee should take a public position on legalizing physician-assisted death).

Identifying the realm or level of ethical analysis is important because the good that is being sought at each level changes, from the good of the individual, to the good of the institution, to the good of society. Because bioethical consensus has been at the individual level, there is a tendency to assume that the same assumptions and conclusions can apply at each level. However, this is not necessarily the case. For example, it may be that physician-assisted death serves the good of some individuals but not the good of the institution; or it may serve the good of the institution but not the good of society.

The Institutional Realm

Ethics committees are much less experienced with ethical analysis at the institutional and societal levels than they are at the individual level. However, institutional ethics is becoming increasingly important and ethics committees are being asked to address these issues. In the past five years, most acute care hospitals have had to think about institutional ethics in terms of policies concerning health care professionals infected with HIV and ways of protecting health care professionals from becoming infected with HIV as a result of workplace exposure. Those ethics committees involved in the development of HIV policies became acutely aware that the analytical approaches that worked well in patient care questions did not lend themselves to questions involving either a conflict between patient and physician interests (for example, whether a patient could be tested for HIV without consent when a health care professional had experienced a significant exposure to the patient's blood) or a conflict between the institution's obligations toward patients and toward staff (for example, whether hospitals could require health care professionals to reveal their HIV status to patients).

In addition, institutions are rapidly discovering the ethical nature of decisions and issues that previously were thought of as financial, administrative, organizational, or human resource questions. Other issues now being discussed with increasing frequency include the allocation of resources in the institution (not only in the planning and budgeting process, but also in the patterns of diagnostic test use and of intensive care admissions and discharges). Another emerging issue is that of futile or inappropriate treatment. Institutions as well as professionals are exploring their rights and duties to set limits that may conflict with the expressed wishes of patients and/or their families for treatment.

Transferring the principles, methods, and priorities from the realm of individual ethics to that of institutional ethics will almost always lead to unsuccessful attempts to resolve institutional problems. When ethics committees move or are asked to move beyond the level of individual treatment decisions, they must seriously consider whether they are the best group to address the problem. Whatever the answer, it must be in cooperation with other groups in the institution. Policies on determination of death by neurological criteria (brain death) require the involvement of neurologists; policies on institutional approaches to HIV testing and health care professionals require cooperation with infectious disease specialists and employee health departments; policies on organ donation referrals in the case of anencephalics may need the involvement of the trustees; policies creating special forms for DNR orders should involve the critical care and medical records committees.

Some specific challenges in this area that *would* be appropriate for the ethics committee to consider (alone or in collaboration with other groups in the institution) include:

- Implementation of legislative enactments such as the Patient Self-Determination Act
- Institutional programs, policies, and structures to address treatment decisions for persons who are permanently unconscious
- Institutional principles and policies concerning futility judgments made by professionals when patients or their families desire treatment
- Criteria for and policy on admission to and discharge from intensive care units

- Decisions to establish special care units
- Strategies to improve relationships among clinical professionals (such as physicians and nurses)

The Societal Realm

One of the most important tasks in doing ethics is to determine which context deserves priority: the individual, the institutional, or the societal. Daniel Callahan argues that it is our failure to move to the societal perspective that has led us down so many blind alleys in American health care. "We have no lasting hope of devising a decent understanding of health — and thus of fashioning a viable healthcare system — unless we learn better how to attend to the social dimensions of health, indeed unless we learn how to shift our priorities sharply in a societal direction."[2] This conflict about level can also be seen in the arguments about whether, if rationing is necessary, it should be done explicitly at the policy level (a societal decision) or implicitly by physicians at the patient level (an individual or institutional decision). Those who favor the first course may argue that this is a societal decision and must be made on that level, whereas those who favor the second course may argue that U.S. citizens cannot tolerate the idea that their society would specifically deprive them of useful health care. Thus, it would be more acceptable to individuals to have the rationing done less explicitly at the individual level, even though it is a societal issue. Also, physicians may resent having the burden of limiting patients' options placed on them.

Ethics committee members are touched by societal ethics as are all members of society. Societal issues are usually appropriate topics for committee education. What is not as clear is whether committees *as committees* (rather than as individuals) should become involved in these issues in a more direct manner. For example:

- Should committees become involved in the political or public policy process by attempting to influence legislation or by persuading voters about legislative initiatives?
- Should ethics committees take public positions about issues such as legalized euthanasia or national health insurance?
- Should the committee's mission be to provide education or to take sides on an issue? (This is a question that relatively few ethics committees have addressed.)

Some ethics committees have testified at state legislative hearings; others have been involved in filing briefs in court cases. One ethics committee briefly became involved in an attempt to change state law concerning HIV testing when the corporate counsel informed the committee that a statutory change would be needed to make the policy acceptable and the committee began to pursue this course with the help of institutional lobbyists.[3]

Ethics committee networks have become involved in shaping public policy in health care (for example, several networks have worked with state and county agencies to create programs in which countywide DNR orders could be recognized and honored by emergency medical technicians; the Midwest Bioethics Center helped to shape the patient self-determination legislation sponsored by Senator John Danforth of Missouri). Ethics committees of professional organizations (physicians, nurses, specialty societies, attorneys, and so on) have been very active in the public policy arena in terms of recommending legislation, issuing "white papers" that are later cited by courts, and influencing public opinion.

The role of hospital ethics committees in this arena is in its infancy (and may stay there). Given the amount of work that needs to be done within the institution itself, and given the largely voluntary work of ethics committee members, it may be that as individual committees, their contribution will bear more fruit at the local level. Furthermore, they certainly risk alienating their hospital communities if they begin to publicly endorse positions that are being vigorously debated in public. In addition, if they actively pursue a lobbying role, they may jeopardize their institution's tax-exempt status if it is a charitable organization (Section 501(c)(3), Internal Revenue Code) or its future budgetary status if it is a public institution (military, Veterans Affairs, or state or county hospital).

However, there are levels here, as well. Ethics committees can educate themselves on political issues, debate them, educate staff and community, try to formulate positions, invite support on a position from other groups in the community, or directly lobby: the lesser stages seem clearly to be valuable. As issues such as active euthanasia move to the political agenda, it would surely be unfortunate if ethics committees considered themselves voiceless *because* the issue had become political. Nevertheless, the addition of a political context makes matters more difficult for ethics committees, as it does for ethicists when they must decide whether they are functioning as educators or as advocates of a position and, if the latter, whom they represent.

Forms of Ethical Analysis

Most of the methods advocated in bioethics are in some way based on the use of rules and principles (deontological ethical analysis) or based on calculating the consequences of various options and their impact on the players or on society (teleological ethical analysis). Following are brief descriptions of some methods currently thought to be helpful in applied health care ethics.

Principled Ethics

The most commonly held view of how ethical analysis in health care should proceed is probably that put forth by Beauchamp and Childress in *Principles of Biomedical Ethics*.[4] Although these philosophers discuss both deontological (principled) and teleological (consequential) ethics, what has been most appealing in their approach has been what is often called the "mantra" of bioethics: "autonomy, nonmaleficence, beneficence, and justice." The application of principled ethics proceeds by determining what principles are at stake or are in conflict in any particular issue and then determining by argumentation (the giving of reasons and justifications) which principle should take precedence.

Thus, in the case of a terminally ill male patient who wishes to forgo treatment but whose physician believes that he should try one more round of chemotherapy with some small chance of success, the case would be analyzed as follows: The principle of *patient autonomy* is in conflict with the principle of *physician beneficence*. The physician has an obligation to urge on the patient that which the physician believes will best serve the patient's health and well-being. The patient, however, has the right to decide whether the burdens and risks of treatment are justified by the possibility of continued life of a given quality. When making a principled analysis in such a case, it could be said that if the patient understands the risks and burdens and benefits of treatment and also understands what will happen if he forgoes all treatment, then he is best situated to decide what course of action is consistent with his own values concerning how he wants to conduct his life and his death. Some might also urge that the patient be able to explain to the physician his reasons for refusing treatment. In this case, the physician has met the obligation of beneficence by *recommending* what the physician thinks is best for the patient; but because patient autonomy is more important, the patient is entitled to decide what course he wants to follow.

In any ethics committee consultation, *patient autonomy* and *beneficence* are used quite consciously and consistently in this manner. Those who have been involved in ethics committees for more than a decade can remember a time when asking what the patient wanted (attending to the value of patient autonomy) was met with perplexed looks and no response, for no one had even thought to ask. Nowadays, it often happens that no one has thought to ask the question while the patient is still able to answer, but the question itself no longer results in perplexity. It is widely understood as an important and appropriate question whose answer is vital to resolving the issue at hand.

This wholesale endorsement of patient autonomy sometimes seems to *require* patients to be autonomous decision makers, even if they would rather not be (as many would not when they are very sick or very uncertain about difficult treatment choices). However, this problem can be resolved by the understanding that one choice of the autonomous patient is to relinquish the right to make decisions, even if that choice means that he or she is turning these decisions over to paternalistic physicians, suspect families, or indifferent courts.[5]

Principled ethics tells us what is important, but it does not, in and of itself, tell us anything about which of two important principles is more important in a given case. We may use consequences or moral intuitions or cultural beliefs to make that decision, but we must explain why those choices are justified. Current consensus is that in treatment decisions patient preference/patient autonomy is the more authoritative principle assuming that (1) the patient understands the situation and is able to communicate and make a judgment based on personal values and (2) the treatment can reach appropriate medical goals, thus making these decisions somewhat easier.

However, most difficult decisions involve patients who do not and cannot have such understanding, and whose prior wishes are either not known or not known in sufficient detail. Principled ethics provides little guidance in these cases, but our reliance on patient autonomy to guide us in individual cases has led us to pursue public policies that stretch out patient autonomy through advance directives such as living wills and durable powers of attorney for health care, or to espouse concepts such as substituted judgment that suggest we are able to figure out what the patient would have wanted, even in the absence of any specific information. It is difficult to know whether these arguments will continue to prevail, given the increasing research data suggesting that patients are reluctant to fill out advance directives and that neither family members nor health care professionals are very good at predicting what the patient's wishes are when such directives are absent.[6]

Clinical Ethics

In 1982, Jonsen, Siegler, and Winslade published a handbook entitled *Clinical Ethics,* in which they presented an alternative method to the Beauchamp–Childress mode of ethical analysis to be used in the clinical setting. This method, too, is based on the use of principles, but it provides a somewhat different way of organizing them. Their methodology, which is as reasonable as the Beauchamp–Childress method of principled analysis, espouses a four-step method:

1. Gather the medical facts and determine all that can be determined about the patient's condition and prognosis.
2. Determine the patient's preferences in the light of those facts.
3. In the absence of knowledge about patient preferences, determine as best as possible what will be the patient's quality of life with and without treatment. This is to be determined from the patient's perspective.
4. Consider the impact of socioeconomic factors on the decision. Socioeconomic factors are described as "the burdens and benefits that fall on parties other than the patient."[7]

Such a method is likely to lead to the same results that principled analysis has, assuming that the patient is capable of making reasoned preferences and that those current preferences are known. However, the results may be rather different when the patient lacks capacity and his or her preferences are not known, which is the more common case. In this scenario, an assessment of the patient's quality of life may lead to conclusions toward which family members or caregivers are unsympathetic. For example, the patient may be suffering or may be experiencing nothing at all (as in the case of the permanently unconscious patient), and his or her care may be burdensome to health care professionals, family members, or society in general (because of its costs). If it is not known whether the patient would want continued care, this analysis could lead to the conclusion that he or she should not receive further care, even if the family or caregivers wanted care continued for their own reasons.

Like Beauchamp and Childress, Jonsen, Siegler, and Winslade endorse the dominance of patient preferences (autonomy) when that is possible. When it is not, however, they espouse an assessment, discussion, and consideration of other factors. Like other methodologies, theirs does not indicate exactly how these other factors (quality of life and socioeconomic factors) are to be sorted out. However, this uncertainty about how to balance or weigh various factors is inherent in most applied ethical analysis. The problem may well be in the use of words such as *weigh* and *balance,* which imply some kind of quantification that is simply not possible. Saying that factors should be *weighed* implies that there is some means of weighing them; however, that *means* is not obvious to anyone or clearly elucidated in any method of ethical analysis.

The form of the clinical ethics methodology is intended to be a strong point because it resembles the way in which physicians are accustomed to "presenting" a patient. However, by now, the autonomy–beneficence–justice mode of principled analysis may be familiar to most physicians, or at least to those health care professionals who have been particularly interested in bioethics.

Feminist Ethics

The work of Gilligan,[8] Noddings,[9] and a number of feminists[10,11] has often been endorsed as a helpful way of looking at applied bioethics. The nursing literature, in particular, has placed considerable emphasis on Gilligan's description of an ethical approach in which the preservation of existing relationships is an important value in resolving ethical dilemmas. Such an approach is distinctly different from that of either principled methods or clinical ethics category consideration, because it rejects the atomized and isolated world view that individualism and patient autonomy encompasses. As a result, patient preferences may not have the same force of argument in feminist ethics as they do in other methodologies.

Although neither Gilligan nor Noddings has written about ethics in medical care (other than abortion decisions), some feminists have tried to apply the argument more specifically to health care ethics.[12] Looking at ethics committees, Sichel argues that a feminist ethics of caring is often part of the ethics committee's deliberations.[13] She uses as an example the case of an incompetent elderly patient whose wishes are known but whose children disagree about what course to follow. She accurately notes that, although the committee will support following the patient's wishes, it will go to considerable lengths and spend considerable time in an attempt to obtain consensus about this course from all the children, believing that it has a duty to care about the family as well as the patient. It would appear that if the patient's wishes were the only important factor, the course of action desired by the patient should be followed immediately, rather than after the children have been persuaded to agree.

A commitment to caring and preserving relationships can also be seen in cases involving seriously ill newborns. Those working primarily within principled analysis would argue that the newborn is entitled to receive any and all medical treatment that will permit it to live, even if its life is of lesser quality than the parents might be willing to accept for their child. Those arguing within the clinical ethics categories might focus instead on whether the child's quality of life, as the child would perceive it, would be sufficiently rewarding to justify continued treatment. These claimants argue that the child should receive treatment if there is the prospect of sufficient benefits to the child (at reasonable cost to others), but that treatment should not be given if there are not sufficient benefits compared to burdens, regardless of parental preference. That is, the decision is based not on the parents' preference or willingness to accept the child into their family but on the infant's quality of life.

Feminist arguments are more likely to focus on decisions for the family as a group in which relationships exist and will continue to exist in the future (for example, what the impact of this child would be on the existing family, including other children) and how these decisions will foster relationships rather than destroy them. Thus, justifications for failing to treat would be more likely to involve parental and family preference about whether and how the newborn could be sustained within existing relationships and whether new relationships could be made that would integrate the child into the family.

Feminist ethics is frequently described in terms of webs or networks (as opposed to principled ethics, which is sometimes characterized as ladderlike). The emphasis is on relationships and connections rather than on isolated individuals. The values of an ethics of caring are frequently voiced in ethics committee discussion, particularly by those who are most cognizant of the relationships that patients have with families and friends and of the impact that the patient's illness has on those relationships.

Casuistry

Jonsen and Toulmin offered yet another view of applied bioethics in their 1989 book, *The Abuse of Casuistry*.[14] This book appeared to be a conscious attempt to refute the methodologies based on principles and had as its source the authors' experience with the National Commission for the Protection of Human Subjects of Biomedical and Behavioral Research. There, they observed that commissioners seldom agreed on why a specific practice was wrong but quite reliably agreed that it was wrong. Clearly, they concluded, the commissioners were using some method other than principled reasoning to determine their judgments. Yet, casuistry, too, relies on principles and rules (as well as a consideration of consequences). Their book attempts to revive casuistry, a historically prominent method of ethical analysis, and to apply it to health care.

In its simplest form, a casuistic analysis assumes that there are *paradigm cases* about which we can all agree as to the right or wrong resolution, even if we have different reasons for our positions. The task of case-based ethics is to create or find paradigm cases and then determine how the case before you is similar to or different from the paradigm case. There is, of course, more than one paradigm case, and so the additional task is to determine to which category of paradigm case a current case belongs. Thus, one might take the case of Mrs. Jones, a woman in a persistent vegetative state, who had specific knowledge of such conditions and had informed her husband that she would never want medical treatment intended to prolong her life should she become permanently unconscious. Wide agreement could probably be obtained that, if Mrs. Jones were found to be permanently unconscious and needed a ventilator to prolong her life, it would be wrong either to start such an intervention or not to withdraw it if it had already been started.

Let Mrs. Jones, then, be the paradigm case. Soon a new case comes up: Mr. Smith, about the same age as Mrs. Jones, same family background, same information about his wishes, and same diagnosis of permanent coma. However, Mr. Smith does not need a ventilator because he is able to breathe on his own. He does need to be fed by tube. If an ethics committee is asked whether clinicians should withhold artificially supplied nutrition and hydration from Mr. Smith, it must ask in what way this new case is different from the paradigm case of Mrs. Jones. Obviously, the difference is that the treatment question now involves nutrition and hydration rather than a mechanical ventilator. For this to be the paradigm case, the question that must be addressed is whether artificially supplied nutrition and hydration are sufficiently similar, in morally relevant qualities, to the ventilator. Or, conversely, we need to determine whether the artificially supplied nutrition and hydration are sufficiently different in morally relevant ways from the ventilator, so that this case cannot be resolved in the same way that the paradigm case of the ventilator was resolved.

What about the case of Ms. Brown? Ms. Brown is not permanently unconscious but is severely demented and has also left a statement that she would not want treatment if she lost her decision-making capacity. Ms. Brown has a severely infected leg, which, if left untreated, could lead to serious illness and ultimately death. Should she be given antibiotics? Is Ms. Brown's case like the paradigm case of Mrs. Jones, or is it different in some important way?

The case-based method advocated by Jonsen and Toulmin is very appealing in many respects. Much of medicine works on this kind of approach, and so it is very familiar to health care professionals. Furthermore, this approach tends to produce answers that seem intuitively correct. However, there are two obvious problems involved in using casuistry. First, ethicists may not agree about what constitutes a paradigm case.[15] Second, there are no clear rules indicating how to determine whether the case is or is not sufficiently similar to the paradigm case whose resolution was accepted as a model. The members of the ethics committee must struggle to obtain a consensus. What casuistry offers is a stance in which to begin ethical analysis. There is something to be said for initially acknowledging that there is something everyone can agree on and then trying to build on that agreement. But the methodology itself does not guarantee that agreement will follow.

Casuistic methodology is frequently heard in ethics committee discussion: "Isn't this case sort of like the one we talked about two months ago?" someone will ask. "No," someone else will reply, "*That* patient told his daughter he'd never want to go to a nursing home." "But that's not the important thing," another member will assert. The casuistic analysis proceeds with a discussion about whether it is similar (or different). For example, suppose the case involves telling the truth to the Jehovah's Witness mother of a child with anemia. The physician believes that if the child's blood count continues to drop, transfusion will be necessary in the future. The physician asks the committee whether the mother should be told *now* that, at that future point, the physician will obtain a court order to provide the transfusion. The proposed resolution may be very different if this case appears to be about truth telling (the physician should tell the truth) rather than about protecting children (the physician should withhold the truth to ensure that the child receives medical care in the interim).

Other Theories of Ethical Analysis

A number of other books have been written describing other methodological approaches to bioethics that may be of interest to ethics committee members. Engelhardt describes applied ethics as a kind of traffic police activity in which everyone drives his or her own set of values, and the only thing that ethical analysis can do overall is provide a set of traffic rules (such as due-process rules) so that people do not run into each other or navigate in excessively hazardous ways that are likely to harm others.[16] Pellegrino and Thomasma discuss the physician–patient relationship (with emphasis on the *relationship*), in which the physician's obligations of beneficence are defined in terms of his or her understanding of the patient's good as it is understood by the patient.[17] Veatch approaches ethical analysis from the assumption that the relationship between physician and patient is based on a contractual obligation in which decisions are made that are mutually satisfying to both parties and in which beneficence is clearly a subsidiary principle.[18] Zaner, very much *unlike* Veatch, emphasizes the physician–patient relationship as one having a moral character in which the patient must trust the physician and the physician must respond to the unique personhood of the patient.[19] Zaner also finds patient autonomy inadequate as the basis for medical ethics and, instead, looks to the moral integrity of both individuals as it is developed through their relationship. Both of these writers have something important to say about the value dimensions of the health care relationship, and familiarity with their arguments can expand ethics committee members' understanding of the complexity of the issues.

Conclusion

There are multiple methodologies for looking at specific moral issues in health care. Each may be more or less helpful in specific cases or issues. Some are more useful for societal policy issues than are others; some provide more insight into institutional questions than do others. But none provides a universally appropriate methodology for ethics committees.

Furthermore, most of these methods are characterized by concepts and insights that are typically present in the vocabulary of ethics committee members, even if the members have never heard of these theories or their proponents. Ethics committee members who have never heard of Beauchamp and Childress or have never attended the Kennedy Institute intensive course in bioethics speak articulately about the importance of finding out about and then listening to the patients' values when it comes time to make decisions. Ethics committee members do struggle to determine how to characterize the patient's quality of life and whether the benefits to a patient are sufficient to outweigh the enormous emotional or financial burden on family members that continued treatment will bring. Ethics committee members do compare cases and ask how this new case is like the old one and how it is different and whether the differences make enough difference. Ethics committee members do talk about the importance of relationships, whether in the context of prolonging a patient's dwindling life just a few more hours or days in order to await the arrival of a traveling relative who needs to say good-bye, or arguing for the right of a longtime companion to speak for an incapacitated patient rather than a relative who has long been absent from the patient's life. Ethics committee members speak of these issues and many more.

In an essay published in 1990, Brody described ethical analysis as "conversation,"[20] and it is this analogy that perhaps most clearly reflects what ethics committee members do most of the time. Brody suggested that if ethics committee members agreed to continue to discuss a case until not one single member believed there was anything left to say that had not been said and understood, the conversation would address in one way or another all the ethical points from the various ethical methodologies that exist. Such a conversation might not be as all-encompassing as Brody proposes if one were to do it with a group of people who had no experience (either formal or informal) with ethical issues in health care, but even then, it would doubtless encompass the major issues. But ethics committees do not consist of individuals who have had neither formal nor informal ethics education. To be educated as a health care professional, and to practice that profession responsibly, involves extensive experience with and sensitivity to ethical issues, even if the experience does not always appear in the language of philosophers.

Those who have participated on ethics committees report that, although discomfort with "ethics" is a familiar companion at the beginning, over time members begin to recognize familiar themes and to translate their personal ethical language into that of bioethics. Michel has pointed out that "the principles, categories, or paradigms are ways of organizing the facts so that we can understand their meaning in a particular situation."[21] By participating in the conversation of the committee, which is surely a conversation of ethics, members join in the larger conversation of bioethics, which has to do with knowing about landmark (or paradigm) cases, understanding common concepts and terminology, and trusting that communication and common sense are good guides to practical decisions. Brody has said that "expertise in medical ethics does not consist in logical skills of argumentation or having access to a particular theory that provides foundational knowledge of ethics. Instead it consists of having attended carefully to the broadest and most inclusive conversations in the area of medical ethics over a reasonable period of time."[22]

What is the methodology of ethics committees? In the authors' experience, it is eclectic, commonsensical, and reasonably informed and systematic. It is quite good enough (especially given the alternative of no committee), as long as members are always willing to question those familiar and currently accepted ideas that seem so obvious. The conversation is ever broadening. Ethicists may accept the importance of patient autonomy and yet accommodate in the conversation those patients who wish to defer to the preferences of others or who live in cultures in which, as a matter of course, others make decisions for them without either consulting with the patients or even informing them. Ethicists may accept "caring" as a guiding light, but may also have to find a way to accommodate a different viewpoint when, for example, family members want children who clearly meet brain death criteria to be maintained for months on mechanical interventions. Ethicists may accept paradigm cases, only to find that, one day, their obviousness no longer seems so certain.

Health care is filled with uncertainty. It should be no surprise that its ethical issues also are characterized by uncertainty. In support of the art of health care, ethics committees can offer the art of ethical reflection as presented in long and sometimes frustrating conversations in which commitment to clear and honest communication, appreciation of the virtues of common sense, and abiding respect for the values of others will stand them in good stead. The richness of the conversation about ethical issues is what draws most people to ethics committees. By realizing that the diversity of the conversation is an inherent part of ethical analysis, committees may find greater confidence in their work and cease looking for an expertise that would not help them if they had it.

Exercises

1. Divide your ethics committee into three groups. Give each group the same case (for example, the brief case below). Then ask one group to analyze the case using the autonomy–beneficence–justice principled method; ask another to analyze the same case using the four-step clinical ethics method; and ask the third group to analyze the case using case-based casuistry (which means they will have to first decide on a paradigm case). After a half-hour or so, have each group share with the others the points they emphasized and their recommendations for the case. Vicki Michel, who developed this exercise for an ethics committee conference in California, found that most groups had a great deal of difficulty staying with a single method (which is information in itself about how ethics committees work), and so committee members should be counseled to stay with their assigned method, even if it is difficult to do so.

    You may want to repeat this exercise with one group emphasizing preservation of relationships, one holding an unrestricted discussion, and one focusing solely on the consequences of various actions. The point of the exercise is to try to stay with a single method, to determine how helpful it is to use a relatively strict methodology, and to judge the impact of different methods on outcome.

    Sample Case

    Mrs. J is a 58-year-old woman who is brought to the emergency department by her son. She is judged to be suffering from sepsis and has very low blood pressure. However, she assures you that (1) she did not want to come to the hospital but did it only to satisfy her son; (2) she does not want to be admitted to either the hospital or to the ICU, where the physicians propose to admit her, because she hated being there on a previous admission; and (3) she has felt the way she does now previously, several years ago, and has medicine at home that she took then and that, if she can go home and take again, will make her feel much better. A psychiatrist determines that she has decision-making capacity. Her son feels that whatever his mother wants is okay with him. The physicians believe that she has a life-threatening condition, though it cannot at this moment be judged an emergency; however, a state of emergency could arise very suddenly and the woman lives many miles from the hospital. The physician has a relationship with Mrs. J developed over several years and thinks that admitting her to the hospital against her wishes may seriously impair the quality of that relationship.

2. Take any well-known case, for example, that of Nancy Cruzan or Helga Wanglie. Assign the roles (physician, family member, nurse, administrator) in the case to members of the committee. Give the principal actors enough time to develop their roles. Then conduct an ethics committee review. Stop the discussion every 5 to 10 minutes to discuss the kinds of reasons that people are giving for their claims. It may help if one or two people do not participate in the discussion but try to keep track of the reasons that are given. Could the participants think of other reasons to defend the action they want to take?

3. Construct a series of arguments you might use to advance your position if you were in the shoes of the patient, the family member, the physician, and the nurse in a particular case. It is particularly helpful if you are not sympathetic to the position that the person is actually taking in the case.

4. Build a utopia. How would you shape your institution if it were to respond primarily to ethical issues? For example, propose a service that your institution does not currently offer but that you think it should. How would you have this service structured so that it would work (mission, staffing, services, responsibility and authority, patient population, financial issues, personnel policies)? Moving out from one-to-one patient care issues will present a different set of problems and possibilities.

Notes and References

1. Beauchamp, T. L., and Childress, J. F. *Principles of Biomedical Ethics.* 3rd ed. New York City: Oxford University Press, 1991.

2. Callahan, D. *What Kind of Life.* New York City: Simon & Schuster, 1990, pp. 104–5.

3. Wenger, N. S., Ross, J. W., and Young, R. T. An ethics committee's recommendations on testing patients for HIV antibodies when health care workers suffer exposure to blood-borne pathogens. *HEC Forum* 3(6):329–36, 1991.

4. Beauchamp and Childress.

5. Some attorneys, however, dispute whether this is legally permissible, although it is surely an ethically viable position.

6. See: Diamond, E. L., Jernigan, J. A., Mosely, R. A., Messina, V., and McKeown, R. A. Decision-making ability and advance directive preferences in nursing home patients and proxies. *The Gerontologist* 29(5):621–26, 1989; Ouslander, J. G., Tymchuk, A. J., and Rahbar, B. Health care decisions among elderly long-term care residents and their potential proxies. *Archives of Internal Medicine* 149(6):1367–72, 1989; Seckler, A. B., Meier, D. E., Mulvihill, M., and Paris, B. E. C. Substituted judgement: how accurate are proxy predictions? *Annals of Internal Medicine* 115(2):92–98, 1991; Tomlinson, T., Howe, K., Notman, M., and Rossmiller, D. An empirical study of proxy consent for elderly persons. *The Gerontologist* 30(1):54–64, 1990; Uhlmann, R. F., Pearlman, R. A., and Cain, K. C. Physicians' and spouses' predictions of elderly patients' resuscitation preferences. *Journal of Gerontology* 43(5):115–21, 1988; Uhlmann, R. F., Pearlman, R. A., and Cain, K. C. Understanding of elderly patients' resuscitation preferences by physicians and nurses. *Western Journal of Medicine* 150(6):705–7, 1989; and Zweibel, N. R., and Cassel, C. K. Treatment choices and the end of life: a comparison of decisions by older patients and their physician-selected proxies. *The Gerontologist* 29(5):615–21, 1989.

7. Jonsen, A. R., Siegler, M., and Winslade, W. J. *Clinical Ethics.* 2nd ed. New York City: Macmillan, 1986.

8. Gilligan, C. *In a Different Voice.* Cambridge, MA: Harvard University Press, 1982.

9. Noddings, N. *Caring: A Feminist Approach to Ethics and Moral Education.* Berkeley, CA: University of California Press, 1984.

10. Holmes, H. B., and Purdy, L. M., editors. *Feminist Perspectives in Medical Ethics.* Bloomington, IN: Indiana University Press, 1992.

11. Sherwin, S. *No Longer Patient: Feministic Ethics and Health Care.* Philadelphia: Temple University Press, 1992.

12. *Hypatia,* a feminist journal, has published two issues solely addressing feminist ethics and health care issues. See, for example, Sherwin, S. Feminist and medical ethics: two different approaches to contextual ethics. *Hypatia* 4(2):57–72, 1989.

13. Sichel, B. A. Ethics of caring and the institutional ethics committee. *HEC Forum* 2(4):243–56, 1990.

14. Jonsen, A. R., and Toulmin, S. *The Abuse of Casuistry: A History of Moral Reasoning.* Berkeley, CA: University of California Press, 1988.

15. For an example of such disagreement, see Ross, J. W. Great moments in medical ethics teaching. *Hastings Center Report* 21(1):2–3, 1991.

16. Engelhardt, H. T., Jr. *The Foundations of Bioethics.* New York City: Oxford University Press, 1986.

17. Pellegrino, E. D., and Thomasma, D. C. *For the Patient's Good: The Restoration of Beneficence in Health Care.* New York City: Oxford University Press, 1988.

18. Veatch, R. M. *A Theory of Medical Ethics.* New York City: Basic Books, 1981.

19. Zaner, R. M. *Ethics and the Clinical Encounter.* Englewood Cliffs, NJ: Prentice-Hall, 1988.

20. Brody, H. Applied ethics: don't change the subject. In: B. Hoffmaster, B. Freedman, and F. Raser, editors. *Clinical Ethics: Theory and Practice.* Clifton, NJ: Humana Press, 1990, pp. 183–200.

21. Michel, V. Effective strategies for approaching ethical issues. In: J. L. Drezner and M. Moore, editors. *Ethical Issues in HIV Care.* Los Angeles: AIDS Project LA, 1990, pp. 13–23.

22. Brody.

4

Ethics Committee Meetings: How They Work

The meetings of ethics committees deserve a great deal of careful attention because they are the very life of a committee. If we want to know what a committee is, and not just what it says or thinks it is, we should examine the life and character of the committee as expressed in its meetings. No single meeting reflects this, but an extended series of meetings—over a period of 6 to 12 months, for example—will mirror how the committee works: who and what really matters, what captures the heart of the group, what gets too little or too much attention, who talks, and who listens. Meetings show whether *interdisciplinary* is merely a catchword or a reality for ethics committees. Thus, in one sense, the way its meetings work reveals the soul of the committee.

Beyond that, meetings are the arena in which the committee takes shape. It is in meetings that we reflect on what we do and assess how closely our work reflects our vision. In them, we generate the ideas and plans we need to improve, and we provide the mutual support and motivation needed to take up anew our service to the institutional community. We can help one another learn what needs to be learned about the field and about the institution the committee serves.

Although this chapter focuses on the regular meetings of all the members, there are many other kinds of meetings that can and should make up the life of an ethics committee. This fuller picture includes emergency meetings, such as prospective case consultation; educational meetings; orientation meetings for new members; and meetings of subgroups or subcommittees, such as a steering committee to assist the chairperson in attending to the committee's needs, a membership/election subcommittee, a subcommittee for developing the educational agenda, a subcommittee for drafting hospital documents and policies, and so forth. Some of these meetings are composed solely of ethics committee members; others may include nonmembers. Often, there are additional educational meetings, which may last an hour, a half-day, or a full day, in the case of an off-site retreat, for example. Meetings may be held at the institution or elsewhere. In some meetings, committee members predominantly listen—in much the same way that participants in a congressional hearing do—and in others, committee members talk and make decisions. In some meetings, invited guests—such as hospital administrators, medical specialists, state legislators or local community officials, and local AIDS organization members—speak on issues of mutual concern.

Each type of meeting has a different purpose and payoff for the committee. Although no one committee will regularly exercise all these options, the wider the range of options, the greater the payoff, providing more opportunities to work with others and learn from one another. Thinking about the ethics committee in terms of meetings—the form they take, who attends, and what is discussed—can be a helpful way to explore ethics committees in terms of both evaluation and future direction.

Planning and Evaluating Meetings

One element common to all meetings, regardless of size and purpose, is planning. Productive, satisfying meetings do not just happen, they are thought out and organized ahead of time. Although we have found a direct correlation between the energy and time spent planning meetings and the meetings' success, in many cases the planning aspect appears to receive less attention than it deserves. One way to focus on planning is to establish a definite time, place, and responsible party for its implementation. Too often, the committee chairperson is left to handle the task on his or her own and, as a result, planning is handled quite casually. Designation of a steering committee to take on this responsibility is likely to be a much more successful method of planning effective meetings.

The Roles of Steering Committees and Chairpersons

Committee meetings tend to be satisfying and productive in proportion to each member's sense of responsibility for what happens in them. If members feel invited and empowered to influence the manner and content of the meetings, this is one sign of a vigorous and healthy committee. There is, however, a need for some person(s) to take special responsibility for coordinating meetings. Rather than giving this task to the chairperson or cochairperson(s) to handle alone, it may be more productive to assign this task to a steering committee consisting of the chairperson and several other members, such as the secretary and the chairpersons of all standing subcommittees or to a group of long-term members. The steering committee's responsibility would be the care and nurturing, planning, and evaluation of meetings. This should result in more energy and imagination being brought to planning. Even a chairperson who is gifted in planning and running meetings will benefit from the support of a team effort.

In addition, if the chairperson shares responsibility for the planning and conduct of the meetings, there is less risk that the committee's success will depend on the efforts of one individual. To be genuinely successful, the ethics committee must be a cohesive group of individuals from different disciplines who work together with mutual respect and responsibility. The chairperson can easily find himself or herself dominating the committee because of the way the committee is structured or because chairpersons are often physicians who dominate the hospital hierarchy. Sharing responsibility with a steering committee is a way of empowering other committee members and keeping the ethics committee from becoming a one-person show. It is also a way of providing continuity and eliminating the risk that the group will feel leaderless when a chairperson must leave the ethics committee. In addition, a team effort demonstrates the multidisciplinary commitment of the group.

Although the steering committee members need to have some understanding of the whole committee's group dynamics, it is even more important that they be able to identify appropriate issues in a timely way, as well as those individuals who can provide educational resources for presentation of those issues. In addition, the steering committee should be able to make decisions on the best way to present a topic, organize a series of issues, or create a smooth transition from the topics of one meeting to those of the next. Steering committee members should have the temperament of educators or an interest in education. Having a steering committee assist the chairperson in planning meetings can bring the strength to this function that its importance demands.

Creating Short-Term Meeting Agendas

The steering committee should plan for the short term by first looking at the next meeting in light of the past meeting. The committee may want to meet for 15 minutes at the end of the regular meeting or schedule a longer meeting within a few days after the regular meeting. However done, this should become a regular practice. This retrospective look at the last meeting asks: Is there anything we can learn from the last meeting that can help next time? Did the meeting bog down; if so, how and why? Where did it work well? What made it work well when it did? Do we have loose ends to pick up next month? Did anything come up that suggests an agenda for the next meeting? This process can be helped by routine meeting evaluations. Some committees have their members spend the last minute of each meeting filling out a brief evaluation of the meeting. The steering committee, or whoever is planning the agenda for the next meeting, takes these evaluations seriously, giving committee members feedback on how they plan to respond to the evaluations. If people are asked to express their concerns, either their concerns should be addressed or the committee leadership should explain why they cannot be addressed.

After the steering committee has evaluated the last meeting, it must then establish the agenda for the next meeting. The committee needs to look at subject matter as well as the process issues that different topics require. Would it help to structure a specific issue with a questionnaire, a role-play, a case presentation, or an article? Who is responsible for guiding the discussion or preparing the materials that will be needed for each item? Who will develop or obtain materials? Thinking in advance about whether the committee will need to refer to former policies or committee documents prepared in other contexts is necessary if the resources are going to be available at the meeting. It is frustrating (but common) to hear the committee chairperson say, "Well, I remember we did something about that last year, but I didn't bring the papers with me, so I don't know."

Most agendas differ greatly in their substantive and process complexity. It is not just that they include different subject matters; it is also that the reality behind the agenda items differs in many significant ways. For example, one issue may be conceptually complex but may create no problems among members (for example, withdrawing ventilators after death diagnosed by neurological criteria). Another issue may have a history of implicit but powerful personal investment and conflict (for example, physicians discussing with nurses the reasons for a patient's refusal of CPR). A third issue may demand imagination and creativity (for example, whether staff can help patients understand the role of advance directives). A fourth may need dogged attention to detail (for example, whether the institution's confidentiality policy adequately addresses concerns of those who enter the hospital under an acknowledged alias). As shown below, a typical agenda does not reveal these significant differences:

1. Review of the minutes of the last meeting
2. Old business: ventilator withdrawal after brain death has been declared
3. New business: policy review concerning confidentiality issues for patients with aliases
4. Case presentation: patients' right to refuse CPR
5. Education: use of advance directives

Thus, it is important to plan the format, or process, of the meeting to fit its particular content and the human realities underlying it. Unfortunately, a common approach used in ethics committee meetings could be characterized as the "announce and wade-in" method: "This confidentiality policy; did anybody have any thoughts about it?" Giving attention to the fit between process and agenda item content can facilitate the effectiveness and satisfaction experienced in a meeting. Tailoring process to substance is a task that ranges from simple to highly complex. If it is relatively simple, the following efforts can help. For each item on the agenda, ask: What is the purpose and expectation concerning this item? Is this for information only, a first read, a matter for extended discussion, a final decision, an issue where brainstorming and imagination are needed? The agenda might include the action mode (for example, for information, brainstorming, first discussion, final approval) along with the time frame allocated. This helps the steering committee develop a realistic work load for the meeting and set parameters for developing an appropriate process to go with each item. It also gives members a fuller sense of what to expect for each agenda item.

Beyond this, committees can develop more sophisticated methods for dealing with the various agenda items. For example, work on a specific topic might be helped by a worksheet or a short attitude questionnaire developed in advance. Group process techniques such as role-playing, storyboarding, and brainstorming can be planned. Devising exercises to help address affective dimensions of issues or to stretch the customary boundaries of topics may be time-consuming, but is often productive. Professionals in the behavioral and social sciences often have the skills needed to address these concerns effectively. The committee can draw on the expertise of its own members, get help from others on staff, or occasionally engage a consultant to help in this regard. This question of fitting the process to the complex human substance of an issue is one that has received little attention in ethics committee literature; it deserves much more. Increased consciousness and skills in this regard will greatly improve the effectiveness of ethics committees.

Doing Long-Term Planning

Long-term planning also deserves attention by the chairperson, steering committee, and committee members. Present tasks are always better understood when they are part of a larger context. It is useful to develop a general year's plan for committee efforts, including educational projects, policies to be addressed, surveys to be conducted, documents to be drafted, and so forth. A specific meeting will have more meaning and coherence if it is seen as part of a larger picture. Some committees use their first meeting of the year to develop a general plan for the year or to present a plan that has been developed by the committee leadership for the members to refine (see figure 4-1 for a sample one-year plan). After the plan is developed, each member should be urged (or even required) to participate in some part of the plan during the year.

By developing a general plan and including committee members in both the general decisions and specific roles, responsibility for the committee's work does not remain solely with the committee leadership. It is important to the committee's success that members have a sense of participation and responsibility, rather than being passive attendants at a series of entertainments or experiences created by others.

The Role of the Chairperson in Conducting Meetings

The chairperson of the ethics committee can be wonderfully effective or dismally counterproductive in nurturing the committee. Because most committees have open-ended agendas, the chairperson can have tremendous influence on the direction the committee takes. For this reason, a chairperson should be chosen for his or her interests and likely level of commitment rather than for his or her profession, position, or title. Also, it is more important that he or she has the skills to run a meeting than to plan one. With the help of a steering committee, meeting planning becomes more of a group effort.

The chairperson needs to have the respect of committee members and should be able to help them feel personally involved and challenged. The most effective chairpersons know how to involve others both at the meetings and through subcommittee work outside the regular meetings. They are enthusiastic about bioethics and its potential contribution to health care institutions. Effective chairpersons also are those who take a broad view in setting committee goals. Committees can get bogged down when members do not experience occasional successes and when they have no sense of direction. The chairperson can use the meeting process to remind members of the committee's mission and can contribute to the planning

Figure 4-1. Sample Ethics Committee Plan for One Year

1. Increase nursing participation in committee discussions.
2. Create brochure in which institutional policies that touch on forgoing treatment are summarized.
3. Conduct three grand rounds for medical staff.
4. Design and conduct survey of awareness of ethics committee activities by staff and physicians.
5. Attempt to develop some method by which committee members can be aware of new legislation that affects ethical issues in health care.
6. Develop half-day orientation program for new members.

process so that members are aware of their successes. For example, one committee, which had presented a series of retrospective cases in which interventions had not worked well, was pleased to have the chairperson schedule a case presentation in which interventions did make a difference—a potentially difficult case that became a good case as a result of educational efforts previously provided by the committee. This helped members remember that it was possible to make a difference in outcomes.

The primary role of the chairperson at meetings should be to ensure that:

- The meeting runs smoothly.
- The agenda is covered.
- Participation is elicited broadly from members.
- Discussions are not dominated by a single individual or group.
- There is some recognized forward motion, however slight.
- The meeting has closure.

Thus, the chairperson should have skills in facilitating communication, managing conflict, and managing the agenda in a timely fashion. Unfortunately, attending to this process means the chairperson is often effectively excluded from the substantive discussions of the committee. This can be a problem if the chairperson has been selected because of his or her greater substantive knowledge and not because of superior skills at managing meetings. Those accepting leadership positions in committees should think carefully about their skills and how they can best apply them. We may tend to think that the chairperson of an ethics committee should be the one who knows the most about the subject or who has the most authority in the institution, but such individuals can fill other important committee roles (especially on the steering committee).

Chairpersons who do not have special skills in running meetings may want to develop formal methods for conducting discussions. For example, most committees operate somewhere between the chairperson's calling on people who raise their hands and his or her allowing people who break into the conversation to speak their piece. A chairperson might experiment with having members who want to speak raise their hands, with the chairperson (or some designated person) keeping a list of those who have so indicated and acknowledging (with a nod) that he or she has noted their wish to speak. The list is then read to the committee and the individuals speak in turn. As the discussion proceeds and others want to say something, they so indicate to the chairperson and are marked down for a turn.[1] If the committee members can live with such formality, there could also be what Kathleen Nolan at The Hastings Center once described as "a point of personal agony," in which a member indicates that he or she *must* speak right away. By creating a list of participants in, and an order to, the discussion, members will have to decide how important it is for them to speak and what is the most important thing they have to say when their turn arrives. But it also provides less aggressive participants an opportunity to speak without having to fight over "air rights."

If the chairperson simply allows discussions to run themselves, the committee becomes the property of those who have a more aggressive or interventionist conversational style. This will also provide those who perceive themselves as more expert (including clinical ethicists and ethics consultants) with a greater opportunity to dominate discussions. By making a list of potential speakers, the chairperson is also better able to realize who is not speaking and then to either solicit their opinions or at least offer them the opportunity to make a comment at the end of the discussion. For example, the chairperson might say at the end of the discussion, "Bill, now that we're coming close to deciding where we go next, do you have any thoughts on anything we might have missed or not considered fully?"

If the chairperson is willing to attend to the process of the meeting, other committee members have a greater responsibility to contribute to the substantive issues. Here, too, it helps if the chairperson has a steering committee whose members feel the weight of this responsibility and can help guide the substance of the discussion, summarize what has been said, be attentive to the areas that have not been addressed, and ensure that the discussion has been thorough, given the time available.

Meeting Times

How a committee handles time is an important element of a committee's culture. The following two issues are critical: beginning and ending meetings on time; establishing agenda time limits.

Beginning and Ending on Time

Inconsistencies with respect to beginning and ending the meeting on time are costly. Starting late reinforces tardy behavior, and it devalues the substance of the committee's work as well as the time of those who made the effort to arrive punctually. Some committees combine the meeting with a meal, and the first 15 minutes are allotted for people to get food and have a few decompression moments. Then the meeting proper begins promptly.

Time is equally important at the end of the meeting. Allowing the meeting to drag on and end in bits and pieces as individuals look at their watches and escape at intervals is demoralizing. Meetings that consistently begin and end as scheduled affirm the worth of both the participants and the issues. This practice also provides a solid basis for tolerance when urgency demands that the meeting run long. However, even such a claim for tolerance should be made in a responsible way. If the discussion is so important that the meeting time needs to be extended beyond the scheduled ending time, the chairperson should tell the committee members as soon as he or she has at least tentatively made that decision. For example, the chairperson might say, "I think it's important that we complete this discussion, and I don't think it's possible to finish it in the next 10 minutes. Therefore, I propose that we extend the meeting an additional 15 minutes, to 8:15." Informing members of what to expect and then conforming to that announcement usually results in most members staying the extra time. However, if the meeting simply continues beyond the closing time, with no announcement, people will begin to escape because they have no way of knowing how long they will be there.

Setting Time Limits for Agenda Items

Establishing time limits for the discussion of agenda items is critical. Most issues could consume the entire meeting time if left without guidance and limits. Setting time limits for agenda items, of course, needs to be done with a degree of flexibility and openness to what is actually happening at the meeting. Rigid adherence to the time announced on the agenda for a given item would not serve the committee well if the substance of the discussion warrants further comment and it appears that the matter could be concluded within a reasonable extension of time. However, allowing each item to consume whatever time and energy it elicits from the committee demonstrates an absence of priorities.

Allotting time limits for the agenda items requires those planning the meeting to consider priorities for the committee's work. If they are wrong and time runs out while the committee is still deeply engaged in the topic, the time can be extended if the chairperson, with the committee's concurrence, judges it appropriate. In this way, the allocation of time is explicitly handled by both those planning the meeting and all members in attendance.

Materials Distribution

Getting materials in a timely way is essential. For example, minutes, policies, patient brochures, and other such documents, as well as educational materials, all require that members have some time for review outside the committee meeting.

Minutes

If a committee genuinely wants to review the minutes and make necessary changes, the minutes should be sent out so that members can read them in a time frame and space that takes them seriously. Shuffling through the minutes for a first viewing after the chairperson asks for their approval hardly qualifies as taking them seriously.

However, it is often the case that, even though the committee sends minutes out in advance, members do not read them until they arrive at the meeting and the chairperson asks whether there is a motion to approve them as written. This suggests that members see no real point in receiving the minutes in advance or even in reading them. If this is the case, the committee may need to discuss why minutes are important. One way that this lack of concern with meeting minutes may be overcome is to use a format for recording them that is helpful to the members from meeting to meeting. Some committees use a format that divides each item on the agenda into three sections: the issue, the committee's action at the meeting, and the committee's disposition or expectation for future action (see figure 4-2).

Such a format is both more compact and more useful to the members than most committee minutes currently are. There could also be a more formal recording of the minutes similar to what most committees currently prepare, and this version could be sent to individuals who did not attend in order to keep them informed. The members who did attend, however, may benefit more from a format that reminds them briefly of what went on last time and where the committee is headed. In addition, the current meeting's agenda can be explained to members as it is moved along in terms of these more succinct minutes of the previous meeting. It is the authors' sense that, if minutes are to provide anything more than an historical record of the committee's activities, committees must begin to experiment with other ways of keeping different kinds of records that will help the members. Some committees formed as medical staff committees do not distribute minutes in advance because of confidentiality concerns. They should be particularly concerned about providing a record for the members that offers useful information in a way that can be discerned quickly.

Textual Materials

The concern for reflective time and space is even more important for texts other than minutes. For example, if the committee needs to review a policy or the text of a patient brochure, the issue is not just getting the text read quickly but also having the time and space to study and reflect on it. Although most members seem to read such materials before the meeting, often they are not sure exactly why they are reading them and what they should be looking for. At the meeting, when the discussion begins to provide a focus, they must look at the text again from this new perspective. If the individuals responsible for presenting the material were to provide members with a review guide that indicated both why the member is to read it and the key points that need to be considered, members could concentrate their personal study of the text. This review guide could then be used to direct the subsequent committee discussion. For example, a review guide for a new policy might include a brief statement saying that "these are the five concerns we tried to address in this document: 1, 2, 3, 4, 5. We see the most significant problems in paragraphs 3, 5, and 9." Or, "The first three pages are unchanged. After that, all changes are underlined and significant changes are in boldface."

The amount of textual material distributed prior to a meeting should be reasonable. When members receive 30 or 40 pages of materials, they are unlikely to read any of them unless planners provide them with some guidance as to what is critical, what is useful, and what

Figure 4-2. Sample Format for Committee Minutes

Issue	Progress	Action
Discussion of DNR orders in surgery.	Committee unwilling to make final recommendation without surgery input.	J. Smith will discuss with chairman of surgery.
Presentation of two cases on pain control.	Discussion emphasized distinction between issues in acute and chronic pain.	Plan further meeting on chronic pain control.

is for information only. Meeting planners should make thoughtful judgments about how much material is necessary for the committee to achieve its goals. Too often, there is a fear that unless everything that is easily available on a topic is distributed, members will not be sufficiently informed. Usually, however, members already have some information about the topic and some mutual education will occur during the meeting, so that total coverage through distributed material is not necessary. Materials distributed in advance should be as concise as possible. For example, if a new policy is being presented, the policy developers should also include an outline of the policy, indicating the salient issues. In one institution, the policy subcommittee indicated in boldface every sentence that had been controversial in the preparation of the policy. Another subcommittee underlined every addition to the proposed policy since the last meeting so that members could focus on the new material. Similarly, when a policy revision is presented, in most cases it is probably more helpful to present only the revised sections. The committee should be able to trust its subcommittee to ensure that the revised section fits within the policy.

Educational Materials

Most committees distribute one or more relevant articles to members at each meeting. It is important to provide time for articles that have been distributed for discussion. Nothing ensures the neglect of articles as effectively as a pattern of running out of time for their discussion. Good results have come from consistently taking time for discussion if articles are sent, setting and sticking to a time limit for discussion, and providing a work page to focus reading and guide discussion. A sample work page includes the following questions:

- What are the article's main points?
- Were the authors' opinions persuasive?
- Are there other articles on this topic that have a different perspective?
- Would this article be helpful to anyone interested in bioethics? Why? Why not?

Some committees assign one or two members the task of leading the discussion on the article. Others ask the members who are to lead discussions to choose the articles themselves.

Methods for Ensuring Member Participation

Like many other aspects of the committee's life, participation deserves attention in two ways. First, it should be a criterion for selecting members. Invitation to join the committee should be extended to those for whom *active* participation is standard operating procedure. Second, attention should be given during the meetings to promoting and facilitating broad participation. Even when members who usually express themselves have been chosen, this quality is a variable across populations—physicians, nurses, other staff, community members—as well as among individuals. One person may speak freely when in the presence of others in the same discipline but reluctantly when in the presence of people from other disciplines. Tannen suggests that women are sometimes more hesitant to speak in public forums than men, even though they may be very articulate in a private setting or when specifically authorized to speak.[2]

Individuals who chair ethics committee meetings need to attend to approaches and processes that make room for the muted voices amid the vociferous. It is especially important to explicitly invite opposing or varying views if a discussion has been swept in one direction by some of the stronger members of the committee. The dynamic of groupthink can be inhibited, if not eliminated, by an invitation such as, "Probably some of us have a different emphasis or viewpoint on this matter." Or more strongly, "Certainly someone sees the matter differently." And even more strongly, "Sarah, can you think of another way that we can look at this?" Repeatedly, this added nudge elicits valuable comments that would have otherwise gone unspoken.

Another method that some committees use to ensure consistent broad participation is to begin each meeting by offering members an opportunity to comment on something they want to share with the committee from their reading, reflection, or experience since the last meeting. This opportunity should be accepted with the understanding that discussion time cannot be allotted to these issues during the present meeting, but could be requested for a future meeting. This technique of offering each member in turn a chance to comment—without immediate discussion—can also be effectively used in discussions of articles, policies, and problems. It gives each participant the chance and challenge to express his or her opinion, makes everyone aware of the full range of perspectives represented in the room on this topic, and avoids a common dynamic that tends to make the first comment the point of reference for much of the following discussion—not because it deserves to frame the question but simply because it was the first point made.

Another mechanism for ensuring participation is voting. This can be on a Lickert-type scale ranging from strongly agree to strongly disagree or simply a yes, no, or abstain. One committee used voting to begin and conclude its discussion of euthanasia. A sample ballot initiative was prepared proposing the legalization of euthanasia under restricted circumstances. The members could vote yes, no, or abstain. The vote was announced and then the prepared discussion was conducted. Toward the end of the meeting, another vote was taken and any changes in attitude and judgment were discussed along with the factors that contributed to these changes. (This is the basis of a method used in some research called the Delphi method: presumably, if the oracle is asked enough times with enough intervening information provided, a group can come to some greater consensus about an issue.)

Such efforts to facilitate participation can provide several elements that are important to ethics. First, they give each individual the opportunity to present his or her own experience and frame of reference without having to immediately react to someone else's; that is, they help us listen to ourselves. Second, they offer the committee a chance to experience the range of positions and opinions, with differing ways to frame the question, before moving into detailed discussion and debate about one or more viewpoints. Third, such measures permit individuals who may feel that their views are unpopular or unlikely to be shared by others to find out that others agree with them or have views that vary from the more common ones. Fourth, they give the group a clearer sense of whether there is consensus, diversity, or strong division on a given issue. The committee should not take such initial positions as determinative in any way. Such statements are what people are willing to say initially. They may not fully reveal their position (they may be willing initially only to test the water), but they are likely to give some indication of the direction in which they are tending. In addition, it is assumed that everyone does not come to a topic with a fixed position. The discussion that is to follow is intended to affect the views of the committee's members. Otherwise, it is a futile exercise. However, without deliberate effort these benefits are less likely and the committee will be poorer for that.

Other mechanisms for enhancing participation include surveys, questionnaires, and evaluations. For instance, some committees keep their attention to meeting satisfaction fine-tuned by providing a quick evaluation sheet at the end of each meeting. The form asks several questions concerning the day's meeting: (1) "What did you like best?" (2) "What did you like least?" (3) "What suggestions can you offer for future meetings?" This type of mechanism tells members that they matter and are responsible for meetings, and it elicits many ideas that would be otherwise lost. However, an evaluation sheet is unlikely to be helpful if it is used only once. Members need to get used to doing this kind of evaluation and they have to believe that doing it will make some difference.

An important way to sustain member interest and vitality in the committee is to consistently invent and plan ways that facilitate broad participation at meetings and throughout the life of the committee. The subject of participation could be valuable as a topic for committee discussion, an item for committee evaluation, and an item for a position statement as part of its foundation documents. (See the section on reinforcement of foundation documents later in the chapter.)

Determining the Functions of the Whole Committee and Its Constituent Parts

As previously noted, an ethics committee is multidisciplinary. It helps if that is recognized in structuring committee processes. *Multidisciplinarity* means that the committee is likely to function best when it mixes and matches a variety of groupings; for example, the whole group, standing subcommittees, ad hoc task forces, work groups of committee members only, and work groups consisting of members and nonmembers. Each such grouping is well suited to perform certain tasks, but ill suited to perform others.

Whole Committee or Subgroup

A few rules of thumb can help a committee take advantage of some group activity matchups and avoid the frustration of others. Members can ask themselves what *their* committee as a whole tends to do well or what it is likely to do well—self-education, evaluation, policy review, brainstorming, educational programs, policy writing, brochure preparation, video projects, event critiques, document preparation, or certain kinds of case consultation. Different committees have different skills and interests. Knowing what the committee members do well and most enjoy should affect the division of labor between the whole committee and its subgroups.

The next question to ask is, What areas tend to be frustrating when attempted by the committee as a whole? Whatever it is, it probably would be better done by a task force or subcommittee. Drafting and/or revising a policy document, an educational/informational brochure, or a questionnaire; framing the questions of a large, complex issue; and developing the schedule for an educational program would all probably be better done in subcommittee, with whole committee participation at various points. Most larger efforts of an ethics committee need both the broad span of whole committee perspective and the focused attention of a smaller group. The secret lies in figuring out which phases of the project need the smaller group (and which smaller group) and which ones need the larger group.

The committee will benefit from explicitly asking this question about a particular issue and arriving at consensus about it. For example, the committee might want to discuss how movement between larger and smaller groups should be orchestrated with respect to policy development. Should the whole committee decide what policy should be written, or should that decision be the prerogative of the smaller group? Clearly, the smaller group will do the drafting, but at what point will the larger committee have input in the process? This can involve a complex set of movements, and failure to clarify who is contributing what can be very frustrating to those on the smaller committee if they perceive that the larger committee is interfering with their work. Conversely, the larger committee may be disturbed if it thinks that the subcommittee is trying to force its position, especially if the larger committee is not sure that the position is representative of the committee as a whole. As one frustrated policy subcommittee chairperson described it: "I don't know whether we're supposed to go and discover a reasonable position for the committee to take on this issue or go and draft a document that represents the position that this committee already has developed but hasn't told us about." In addition, clearly allocating responsibilities makes it easier to keep the committee from becoming frustrated and wasting time when it is apparent, for example, that the committee is wordsmithing a document instead of offering suggestions for the task force to take back for their further efforts. In general, it is never helpful for the whole committee to decide how to word a specific text. The committee can determine what general position it wishes to take, and then committee members can individually suggest, in writing, specific language to capture that position. However, the latter action should not be confused with the former as a committee responsibility. If members do not care enough about wording to write down suggestions they want the subcommittee to consider, the members' concerns about language need not be taken very seriously. If the larger committee begins to engage in wordsmithing, the chairperson should call a halt to this activity. It is remarkable how easily committee members become engaged in this kind of activity and how irritated they are after the fact, as if it had been forced on them by others.

The monthly meeting should include interaction between the whole committee and its various subcommittees and work groups. Besides providing reports to keep the members abreast of the work in progress, the subcommittees can use this fuller forum to test their ideas and to generate fresh ideas from the many perspectives represented in the larger committee.

Education as Process

Given the importance of education for ethics committees—for themselves and as a service to their publics—a good adage might be that no committee should meet without allotting some time for education. The full task of self-education for the committee requires more time and flexibility than the monthly meeting offers, but certain discrete issues can be addressed during the monthly meetings. These include, for example:

- The special needs of new members for general orientation
- The specific needs of the policy committee for its policy-writing work
- The expanding body of court/legislative reality with which to keep pace
- The escalating phenomenon of patients being morally injured by a hurried, stressed, and financially constrained health system

For this segment of its monthly meeting, the committee should aim for consistent but varied attention to education. In the course of a year's time, this educational effort should cover a wide range of topics, dimensions, and methodologies. Articles from leading journals are important, but so too are short stories and poems about health care that go beyond forgoing treatment to include such diverse topics as the meaning of professionalism, patients' experiences of health care, legislative reform of health care, ethics research, and theories of case consultation.[3] Expanding the horizons of committee members can be done by reading, viewing a video, participating in role-playing exercises, or inviting guests to share their perspectives (for example, persons with AIDS, Jehovah's Witnesses or Christian Scientists, surrogate mothers, feminists who have special interests in health care issues, and so forth). If a committee member has a special interest in bioethics, that person might be asked to speak a few moments on important issues that have arisen in the past month involving ethical issues in health care (for example, legal cases, medical advances, important journal articles). The purpose of the educational segment of the meeting is to *inform*. It is important that committee members feel they are part of the bioethics conversation.

But the educational segment of the meeting can also be used to sharpen analytic skills and promote team building and group cohesion; for example, asking members to identify central ethical issues in detailed case vignettes can help develop common vocabulary and similar approaches to case review. The committee will benefit if education, a very broad field of reality for ethics committees, is not left to chance. A considerable planning effort is needed to provide the right balance of different topics and approaches and to evaluate these efforts. This will make up a substantial part of the steering committee's or the educational subcommittee's responsibility for planning meetings.

Education should be substantively relevant. However, relying solely on a format of readings and lectures will probably be counterproductive to the committee's morale. Members have volunteered their time to be on this committee because they wish to participate. Learning, too, should be participatory.

Reinforcement of Foundation Documents

From time to time, it is healthy for the committee to turn to a fuller development of its foundation documents. This can take the form of an update of its bylaws or purpose statement (for example, to make education its primary objective, to expand its range of activities to include advocacy for public policy, to delete an activity now assumed by another group, and so on). Alternatively, it may involve the development of further statements, policies, or positions that relate directly to the committee itself.

One committee developed a letter emphasizing meeting attendance. This letter is used in two ways: one version of the letter is sent to prospective new members of the committee; a second version (see figure 4-3) is used as a reminder to current members when attendance becomes a problem. Another committee focused on the issue of communication within the committee and decided to develop a brief consensus statement on this topic, which members included among their foundation documents (see figure 4-4).

These are ways that ethics committees have continued to revise their self-identity and formulate some newly identified aspects. A number of topics could be addressed by a committee in its foundation documents, including time management, participation, education, advocacy, and so on. Each committee's history and experience will be its guide in this regard.

Figure 4-3.   Sample Letter on Attendance Policy

Dear _____

As we have been evaluating our committee's performance, an important issue has emerged that deserves special attention—the question of consistent attendance at our monthly meetings. Such consistent attendance is critical for an ethics committee—and perhaps different in this respect from some other hospital committees—for several reasons. Many committees can simply rely on the shared assumptions and already-developed expertise of their individual members. The Ethics Committee needs to develop a shared universe of discourse—an explicit consensus on definitions, principles, distinctions, and methodology of ethics. To do this, we will need to spend consistent time together accumulating this shared information and expertise. Beyond this, the maturing of the Ethics Committee requires that it grow as a community of respect and trust. Such growth is promoted by a common commitment, time spent together, communication with one another about sensitive and complex issues, listening to one another's views, and supporting and challenging one another's perspectives. Inconsistent attendance at committee meetings stunts the growth of the committee on two levels: as a community of shared ethical expertise, and as a community of respect and trust.

We understand that limited absences are inevitable. But our goal is to make them as few as possible, for the reasons given above. On those rare occasions when you cannot attend, it will help the committee if you send an alternate in your place. We are developing a list of alternate members who have already had experience on an ethics committee. You can choose an alternate from this list. We suggest that you choose someone whose expertise is close to your own. In order to enhance the effectiveness of our ethics committee, we will be acting as follows: when a member has been absent twice, without sending an alternate, the member will be contacted to clarify her or his intention of continuing to serve on the committee. Further absences by a member, without alternate attendance, after this contact will be assumed to indicate the intention to no longer serve on this committee.

We want to emphasize that our insistence on this question of attendance flows from the very nature of doing ethics and the demands of serving the hospital community as an ethics committee. Should you have any questions or comments please contact us.

Figure 4-4.   Consensus Statement on Internal Communication

The quality of communication goes to the very heart of ethical deliberation. Because the key characteristics of communication that enhance ethical reflection are not always well understood and because patterns of hospital communication sometimes go contrary to such key characteristics, we judge it helpful to explicitly state some of our working assumptions. Explicit discussion of our communication patterns and their periodic formal evaluation are important.

- First-name use is our norm at committee meetings because it symbolizes and builds collegial respect.
- In order to resist groupthink, opposing points of view are not only tolerated, but also should be invited if they are not forthcoming.
- Domination of the discussion by a few hinders adequate discussion.
- Although each person is responsible for his or her own active participation, inviting the comments of those who have not spoken on an issue often elicits important content.
- Silence for reflection is an essential part of the communication process.

Ethics Committees as Communities of Respect and Trust

Effective ethics committees are not simply a selection of people from different professional backgrounds who meet in a hospital at regular intervals. If committee members are to function well, they must become a cohesive group; they must be able to relate well to one another as individuals and to work together as a team. In other words, the committee must gel.

There is voluminous literature on groups—phases of development, process, dynamics, purposes, and so on.[4] Scarcely any of this sociological and psychological wisdom has been applied to the ethics committee phenomenon. This is unfortunate because ethics committees can certainly benefit from established knowledge about groups. It is likely that the study of ethics committees as groups and communities will grow as academics become more interested in the committees and obtain access to them. It is also likely that the existing knowledge about groups and communities will be applied to ethics committees by those serving on the committees.

As an example of how extant knowledge from behavioral science might be applied to the ethics committee movement, we will take several key ideas from Carl Rogers and explore their implications for ethics committees and how they spend their time at meetings. Rogers points to two elements characterizing groups that promote growth for participants and enhance the effectiveness of their service:[5-7] unconditional positive regard and empathic understanding.

Unconditional Positive Regard

Unconditional positive regard indicates a fundamental respect for other people, a recognition that, whatever the differences of education, function, position, or opinion on a given issue, all are basically equal as human beings, deserving both recognition and respect. This basic respect grounds human interaction on all levels. In case of doubt, it trumps all other considerations. It does not mean that one person has only positive judgments about another or that one person views another's abilities and behaviors through rose-colored glasses. People can still disagree, be angry, or be impatient with one another. It does mean, however, that underlying the interaction of any two people in the group is the recognition and affirmation of each other as equal human beings.

Two rules of thumb exist about unconditional positive regard. First, in adults, respect for others is present or absent in varying degrees and not easily changed. Therefore, it is first and foremost a question of selection, not education. Thus, a central concern in selecting members of the ethics committee should be to pick persons who habitually exhibit such respect. Second, such respect can be enhanced or diminished to some extent by the way ethics committee members spend their time at meetings. The better members know each other as individuals and the less dependent they are on knowledge of roles, functions, professional competencies, or positions on specific topics to determine attitudes, judgments, or responses, the better able the committee will be to provide a deepening basis for unconditional positive regard.

Having a deeper knowledge of one another as individuals certainly does not guarantee unconditional positive regard, but the further from this members are, the more they must rely on the stuff of elites and hierarchies—skills, roles, positions, and titles. Ethics committees should therefore spend time not only on honing analytic skills and acquiring new intellectual tools and further factual information, but also on getting to know one another as individuals.

Some committees provide for this in various ways. For example, having meetings at the end of the workday—from 5:00 p.m. until 8:00 p.m.—provides time for dinner together as a social event rather than a working meal. Some of these types of meetings begin with a brief "social rounds" where each person is invited to share a personal item of interest that need not relate to ethical matters but simply honors the fact that each person comes to the meeting with his or her own personal identity. Others offer each member a chance to share a personal observation on an issue or experience of ethical concern. This is not the time to take up these issues in detail (although a specific issue might well be pursued either because it relates directly to already-planned business or because there is enough room on the planned agenda to accommodate its discussion). Such items can simply be offered for information or as a possible or petitioned subject for future attention. An annual ethics committee all-day retreat can also provide the time and setting for a deeper personal presence.

There are specific exercises that the committee can take time for as part of regular meetings, at special educational sessions, or as part of an annual retreat day. Such exercises specifically intend to deepen the feeling of community and to enhance unconditional positive regard. (For example, see the exercises at the end of this chapter.)

Empathic Understanding

Empathic understanding refers to seeing reality from another's point of view. Again, some people are more open to this than others; this is a desirable characteristic in the selection of ethics committee members. Activities can be built into ethics committee meetings that enhance the opportunity for and depth of the members' empathic understanding. Rather than having a nurse, physician, or attorney comment on a particular case, the committee might be better served by hearing a presentation of the larger context from which these particular comments emerge. That is, the nurse or physician could be asked not simply to give a personal response, but also to consider why he or she has that response; in other words, what it is particularly about his or her personal life or professional training that has led to this view. The ethics committee's time could then be spent exploring these other significant frames of reference.

Committees might also invite different individuals to share their professional perspectives on some of the issues committees grapple with. For example, a physician, an attorney, a nurse, and a social worker on the committee could each be asked to prepare a presentation on a specific case. They could share the mind-set they bring, past experiences that have shaped their approach, how their professional training has shaped their views, and how they think their views differ from those in other professions. This could be structured so that all four make a presentation at the same meeting, two present at each of two consecutive meetings, or each one gives a presentation on the same case at each of four consecutive meetings, with another member of the committee providing running commentary on any differences.

These exercises help committee members view familiar issues from different vantage points. Such approaches should not be limited to professional perspectives, but should also include gender, ethnic, cultural, and religious differences. The committee might ask two men and two women to reflect on a single issue, or ask an agnostic, a Christian, and a Muslim. A Jehovah's Witness could be invited to a meeting to explain the meaning of the prohibition on receiving blood and blood products, or a Christian Scientist could explain how his or her religion views its obligations toward children with respect to health care. Individuals from Asian–Pacific cultures or Middle Eastern cultures might talk about the role of consent to medical treatment in their culture. Cultural anthropologists could describe that field's contribution to an understanding of other cultural views. The committee could even invite two members who believe that the present practice of abortion should be changed and two others who believe that it should remain as it now is, or individuals could be invited to present their personal experience.

The goal is not to provoke heated discussion in the manner of a talk show, nor even a cool, rational debate. The ideal is temporary suspension of a desire to persuade or convert. Peaceful listening and contemplating reality from another's point of view is the purpose. Members can return to their own positions later, at which point debate and attempts to persuade can take place.

Conclusion

The success of a committee's meetings can be gauged by the answers to some simple questions. Do members attend? Do they come on time? Are discussions lively? Are there moments of humor as well as moments of seriousness? Do people continue to talk about issues discussed in the meeting after it is over? Are people eager to belong to the committee?

Most committees have reasonably good meetings, and some have meetings with great stretches of time in which one member appears to be lecturing the others. For all committees, there is some variance. However, all ethics committees could benefit from greater attention to the conduct of their meetings. Each committee might develop an instrument for periodic evaluation of its meeting activity. Such an evaluation might include many of the issues discussed in this chapter; however, the key is for each committee to give enough thought and imagination to its own expectations of meetings in order to tailor its own instrument of review and self-renewal.

Exercises

The following exercises are examples of team-building activities that can be part of the reflection of ethics committees. After allowing time to complete the first four exercises privately, individuals can share their ideas with one other person, a small group, or the whole group, as judged appropriate. There is extensive literature on this subject as well as workbooks containing exercises for a range of objectives.

1. List on a piece of paper three desirable characteristics of the following:
   - Physician
   - Nurse
   - Patient
   - Administrator

2. Write:
   - An ideal about health care that you once held dear but that you have changed
   - An ideal about health care that you had early on and that you hold equally or more strongly today

3. Rank-order the following roles by importance for your own self-identity:
   _____ Woman/man
   _____ Nurse/physician/attorney/other professional
   _____ Husband/wife
   _____ Father/mother/son/daughter
   _____ Other

4. Who I am today has been greatly influenced by:
   _____ person(s)
   _____ event(s)
   _____

5. Write (anonymously) two things you hoped the committee would provide for you and two things you thought you had to offer the committee. (The whole committee could then discuss whether members think these qualities/concerns are things the committee can and does offer and that the committee needs.)

6. Write down your primary satisfactions and frustrations with the committee. Put everyone's answers on a single sheet and bring them to the next committee meeting for discussion.

Notes and References

1. This method is used at group projects conducted by The Hastings Center.

2. Tannen, D. *You Just Don't Understand.* New York City: Ballantine Books, 1990, pp.74–95.

3. These four volumes (two of poems and two of short stories and essays) are an excellent source of imaginative material for discussion: Paige, N. M., and Alloggiamento, T., editors. *Vital Signs: The*

UCLA Collection of Physicians' Poetry. Los Angeles: UCLA School of Medicine, 1990; Mukand, J., editor. *Sutured Words: Contemporary Poetry about Medicine*. Brookline, MA: Aviva Press, 1987; Mukand, J., editor. *Vital Lines: Contemporary Fiction about Medicine*. New York City: St. Martin's Press, 1990; and Reynolds, R., and Stone, J., editors. *On Doctoring: Poems, Stories, Essays*. New York City: Simon & Schuster, 1991.

4. Hackman, J. R., editor. *Groups That Work (and Those That Don't): Creating Conditions for Effective Teamwork*. San Francisco: Jossey-Bass, 1990; Zander, A. *Making Groups Effective*. San Francisco: Jossey-Bass, 1982; Tubbs, S. L., editor. *A Systems Approach to Small Group Interaction, Third Edition*. New York City: Random House, 1988; and Cummings, L. L., and Staw, B. M., editors. *Leadership, Participation, and Group Behavior*. Greenwich, CT: Jai Press, 1990. For group process literature that focuses on conflict resolution, see: Fisher, R., and Urey, W. *Getting to Yes*. Boston: Houghton Mifflin, 1981; and Moore, C. W. *The Mediation Process: Practical Strategies for Resolving Conflicts*. San Francisco: Jossey-Bass, 1986.

5. Rogers, C. *On Becoming a Person*. Boston: Houghton Mifflin, 1961.

6. Rogers, C. *On Encounter Groups*. New York City: Harper and Row, 1970.

7. Rogers, C. *Personal Power*. New York City: Dell Publishing Co., 1977.

5

Education for Ethics Committees: What to Learn and How to Teach

Although it is generally assumed that the main activity of ethics committees is case consultation, many argue that the real function—the *raison d'être*—of ethics committees is to provide ongoing education on ethical issues at every level of health care—for the committee itself first and then for the community.[1] Ethics committee education is sometimes perceived as a matter of establishing and communicating expertise, but it is better understood as an activity that enables health care professionals and patients and their families to participate in health care more effectively and with greater personal satisfaction.

In the early days, ethics committees frequently began as study groups, meeting regularly to read pertinent articles or books such as the reports of the President's Commission. In more recent years, however, committees have formed more rapidly and education of that sort has become rare. It is more common today for ethics committee members to be chosen and given a packet of readings or to be invited to a two-hour orientation session. Unfortunately, the readings are seldom removed from their packets and there is little learning as a result of the quick orientation. It is not uncommon to find members of ethics committees who do not understand the difference between a patient who has suffered whole brain death and one who has lost all neocortical function (referring to both as "brain dead"); who are unsure why a patient with a do-not-resuscitate (DNR) order is being considered for surgery or intensive care unit (ICU) transfer; or who say that treatment cannot be withdrawn once it has been started. Members should be informed at the time of their joining the committee that they are expected to study the issues with which the committee deals.

How Much New Members Should Know

Many who believe ethics committees should and do exert considerable power and influence in the hospital are deeply troubled by the committees' lack of bioethics knowledge. They may (and do) say that committees must be much more expert in the literature and concepts of bioethics if they are to be taken seriously, and because they are no longer in their infancy, ethics committees cannot excuse their lack of knowledge on that account.

Different Levels of Knowledge

The position that committees need to have expert knowledge of bioethics seems to miss the defining quality of ethics committees, however. They are multidisciplinary committees whose members come together to provide an environment in which conscious and reflective consideration can be given to significant and often ambiguous value issues in patient care. The arena in which they work, called bioethics, has become a discipline in itself in recent years, but it is both inappropriate and unrealistic to expect each member to bring expertise in bioethics in addition to the expertise of his or her own discipline. Over time, all committee members will learn more about the discipline of bioethics, but they do not need to start with that knowledge. They need to start with an interest in how patient and professional values are lived out in daily acts in health care facilities, a tolerance for ambiguity, and a willingness to commit time to learn more about this new field.

Furthermore, all members need not have the same level of knowledge about bioethics, any more than all members need to have the same level of knowledge of neurology or nursing practice or social work techniques. Members must use one another as resources, but they must also be conscientious about acknowledging what they do and do not know.

A Culture of Trust

It should be easy in an ethics committee for members to acknowledge their lack of knowledge about a particular area outside their own field. However, in a culture in which knowledge is power, admitting to a lack of knowledge may feel very much like admitting weakness. Ethics committee chairpersons, in particular, should be observant about whether committee members can and do ask to have facts, concepts, and distinctions explained to them and whether the committee atmosphere encourages such questioning. For example, when a member confuses whole brain death and neocortical death, does the committee simply step on the confused member by saying, "Well, PVS isn't brain death. If you're brain dead, you're legally dead." Does the member say, "Wait a minute, please explain the difference to me"? Does anyone else say, "Wait, we need to make sure that everyone understands these terms in the same way"? More often than not, members who are unsure or confused are left to learn on their own, picking up the pieces as best they can along the way.

Continuous Learning

If committees do not require members to have a level of education about bioethics prior to becoming members, committees must conscientiously work to educate those members in the course of their time on the committee. In undertaking group responsibility for teaching one another a common body of knowledge, the ethics committee can demonstrate the kind of teaching and learning that should be a model for any moral community. Furthermore, this kind of teaching and learning helps produce a more cohesive group.

One of the great risks of ethics committee education is the furtherance of the idea that ethics amounts to nothing more than the sharing of opinions and that all opinions are equally valid. Although it is surely true that respect is owed to every person's right to have opinions, this does not mean that all opinions are equally valid. In fact, everything is *not* a matter of opinion. Whether a patient has a specific illness is not usually treated as a matter of opinion, even though physicians may disagree about what illness the patient has. Whether the patient has appendicitis is a matter of fact in ordinary language. Whether neurological criteria for brain death are met is, perhaps, a matter of neurological judgment and opinion, but the opinions of a poet and those of a neurologist on this topic are not equally valid. There are spheres of knowledge in which, at least, there is agreement about facts, even if the agreement is only a convention and the "facts" are only previously agreed-to definitions.

Bioethical Consensus

Similarly, there are bioethical "facts" that committee members should all know, if not before they become members at least within a year or two of their membership. These are not facts in the ordinary sense but, rather, judgments and values for which there is general consensus in society. Despite the fact that this is a multicultural society that recognizes many values, it is still possible to discern some areas where there is very broad consensus.

Even where consensus exists, there may be exceptions. Or the consensus may evaporate in the face of new circumstances or understandings. For example, current consensus is that life-sustaining treatment decisions (either to provide or to forgo) should reflect the patient's or surrogate's wishes. However, many are beginning to draw back from that consensus to the extent that it requires providing treatment for permanently unconscious patients. Thus, members must realize that consensus on many if not all of these areas may dissolve as the field develops, as society changes, and as research provides us with greater empirical understanding. One version of the "bioethics consensus" (from an ethical perspective) follows:

Bioethics Consensus Statements

1. The goals of medical care are to cure disease, restore function, eliminate suffering, and prevent illness.
2. The competent and informed patient has the right to refuse any form of treatment, regardless of whether he or she is terminally ill.
3. If a patient is to give informed consent or refusal to treatment, he or she must have decision-making capacity, must have the information about the treatment that a reasonable person would need to have to make a decision, must be able to comprehend the information, must know treatment alternatives and the risks and benefits of all treatment options, must know the implications of refusing all treatment, and must be able to act without coercion.
4. For a patient to have decision-making capacity, he or she must be able to understand the need for treatment, the information given about treatment alternatives and the implications of receiving or refusing treatment, and must have the ability to relate that information to personal values and then to communicate a decision.
5. A diagnosis of mental illness does not by itself justify a judgment that the patient lacks decision-making capacity.
6. The physician has a duty to recommend the course of treatment that in his or her judgment reflects the patient's best interests.
7. When a patient refuses treatment, the physician should understand the patient's reasons for refusing treatment (even though he or she need not agree with those reasons), especially if the refusal will, in the physician's judgment, lead to serious consequences for the patient.
8. If a patient lacks decision-making capacity, a family member or significant other may act as the patient's surrogate.
9. If a patient's wishes about treatment are known, they should be followed; if they are not known, an attempt should be made to determine what the patient would probably have wanted. If that cannot be determined, the decision should be based on the patient's best interests as perceived by family and physician.
10. A best-interests standard does not attempt to assess what the patient wants but rather, from an objective perspective, tries to weigh burdens of treatment and continued life against benefits of treatment and continued life. Any quality of life consideration, however, is to be assessed from the patient's perspective (for example, the patient's perceived experience of burden and benefit).
11. Parents have a right and a duty to make treatment decisions for their children and may be presumed to be acting in their child's best interests. However, it is generally inappropriate to forgo a child's life-sustaining treatment if refusal is based solely on the child's physical or mental handicaps. Decisions should reflect the child's best interests rather than the family's.
12. Similar cases should be treated similarly.
13. There is a psychological difference but no moral difference between withholding and withdrawing treatment under the same circumstances. It is more reasonable to try a treatment and then stop if the treatment does not achieve the patient's desired goal than to withhold the treatment on the grounds that it might not achieve the patient's desired goal.
14. Treatment recommendations should clearly articulate the goals of treatment so that patients/surrogates can be clear as to whether treatment meets their desired goals.

15. Advance directives are helpful in encouraging dialogue among patient, family, and physician about the patient's values and preferences with respect to treatment until such time as they are no longer able to make decisions. Such discussions should not depend on characterizations such as "heroic" or "extraordinary" or "ordinary" treatment because these terms are not amenable to specific definition. Written directives are not ethically more important than oral directives.

16. Rationing decisions should not be made by individual physicians for individual patients. The rationing of health care (decisions about limiting availability of medical care to individual patients) should be explicitly addressed at the policy level, whether at the institutional, professional, or governmental level.

17. Patients may want to use economic factors in making their own decisions, but surrogates' use of economic factors in making decisions for others is controversial.

Do ethics committee members agree with these statements? Are these statements consistent with their professional values? With the institution's mission? Often, physicians have never consciously thought about the goals of medicine and so there may be considerable disagreement as to whether these statements accurately reflect what the physicians intuitively judge to be appropriate. Nurses may understand the goals of health care differently than physicians. In trying to formulate a statement that members agree represents *this hospital's* view of its goals, both professional and individual differences will arise. This can be an effective means of educating members at a very basic level about the values they hold and the values they believe that others hold.

There are many ways to reach this initial level of education about bioethics. For example, it may be helpful for the committee to have all its members make a list (anonymously) of things they do not know or understand about bioethics, and these lists can be used systematically to upgrade members' knowledge. A committee may even want to test members (again, anonymously) to see whether they all have a common understanding of language and concepts. A sample "test" is included in the exercises at the end of this chapter. The point of such a test, however, should never be simply to find out what members know. It is not a test of their knowledge conducted in order to judge them; its purpose is to identify areas in which the committee needs to provide education, often through discussion.

Education for Long-Term Members

Ethics committee members who remain interested should continue as committee members for extended periods. Given the amount of special education that members need to obtain, it makes little sense to be continually educating large numbers of new members at basic levels. After several years of both committee-directed and individual-directed education, committee members should have a broad knowledge of bioethics. Many committee members are able to enroll in intensive seminars or college courses in bioethics, whereas others are more dependent on what the committee can provide. (Some committees have been able to provide stipends for members to attend ethics conferences, at least paying for their registration fees.)

For committees interested in providing their members with a comprehensive education program over the long term, the following is a suggested content outline:

Proposed Education Program for Ethics Committee Members

I. Philosophical Principles and Ethical Analysis
   A. Ethical theories and principles
   B. Nature of professional ethics—altruism, patient advocacy, duty to treat
   C. Ethical analysis and personal opinions
   D. Relationship between autonomy and beneficence; scope of autonomy
   E. Beneficence, nonmaleficence, and the nature of medical judgments about appropriate treatment

    F. Justice arguments with respect to individual cases and at the policy level; public policy implications

    G. Implications of different ethical theories and modes—principled ethics, consequentialist arguments, feminist ethics, narrative ethics, casuistry, Brody's "conversational ethics"

    H. Religious perspectives on health care ethics

    I. Applications of ethical theory and religious principles to case review and policy writing

II. History of Bioethics (and Ethics Committees) over the Past 20+ Years

III. Brain Death, Neocortical Death, and Related Issues

    A. Clinical and legal definition of brain death

    B. Difference between whole brain and neocortical death

    C. Physiological and ethical implications of neocortical death

    D. "Diagnosability" of neocortical death

    E. Relationship of personhood argument to neocortical death

    F. Organ donation—request and consent for, declaration of death

IV. Forgoing Treatment

    A. Legal status of refusing treatment—landmark cases and state interests

    B. Forms and function of advance directives

    C. Surrogate decision makers for patients without decision-making capacity

    D. Medical determinations of incapacity versus legal determinations of incompetency

    E. Withholding/withdrawing distinction

    F. Ordinary/extraordinary/proportionate/disproportionate distinction

    G. Religion-based refusals of treatment

    H. Nutrition and hydration as treatment

    I. Seriously ill newborn treatment standards—disability and justice

    J. State interests in preserving life

    K. Relevant hospital policies

V. Public Policy and Other Principled Issues

    A. Informed consent requirements (content versus documentation); application to HIV testing

    B. Confidentiality—patient information of sensitive or general nature (access to, duty to warn/protect threatened third parties, disclosure to families and friends, legal exceptions)

    C. Truth telling and therapeutic privilege

    D. Medical treatment of involuntarily committed psychiatric patients

    E. Consent to innovative or experimental treatment

    F. Continuity of care (from hospitals to nursing homes, in particular)

    G. Euthanasia (active—voluntary, nonvoluntary, involuntary)

    H. Relationship between law and ethics

VI. Ethics Committee Functions and Obligations

    A. Mission of the committee and the hospital and the hospital's relationship to all committee functions

    B. Confidentiality of information

    C. Patient/family/surrogate access to the committee

    D. Evaluation of ethics committee work

A suggested list of books and journals that will provide a basic bioethics education is shown in figure 5-1.

Sources and Forms of Ethics Committee Education

Some ethics committees require their members to obtain some level of formal education, usually in the form of a specific course offered by a local college. Some ethics committee networks organize such courses, in which case individual ethics committees may be involved

Figure 5-1. Recommended List of Materials for a Basic Bioethics Education

Books

Arras, J. D., and Rhoden, N. K. *Ethical Issues in Modern Medicine.* Mt. View, CA: Mayfield Publishers, 1989.

Callahan, D. *What Kind of Life: The Limits of Medical Progress.* New York City: Simon & Schuster, 1990.

Deciding to Forego Life-Sustaining Treatment, The President's Commission for the Study of Ethical Problems in Medicine and Biomedical and Behavioral Research. Washington, DC: U.S. Government Printing Office, 1983.

Defining Death, The President's Commission for the Study of Ethical Problems in Medicine and Biomedical and Behavioral Research. Washington, DC: U.S. Government Printing Office, 1981.

Fox, R. C. *Essays in Medical Sociology.* New Brunswick, NJ: Transaction Books, 1988.

Jonsen, A. E., and Siegler, M., and Winslade, W. H. *Clinical Ethics.* 3rd ed. New York City: Macmillan, 1992.

Kane, R. A., and Caplan, A. L., editors. *Everyday Ethics: Resolving Dilemmas in Nursing Home Life.* New York City: Springer Publishing, 1990.

Katz, J. *The Silent World of Doctor and Patient.* New York City: The Free Press, 1984.

Kilner, J. F. *Who Lives? Who Dies? Ethical Criteria in Patient Selection.* New Haven, CT: Yale University Press, 1990.

May, W. F. *The Patient's Ordeal.* Bloomington, IN: Indiana University Press, 1991.

Murray, T., and Caplan, A. C., editors. *Which Babies Shall Live? Humanistic Implications of the Care of Imperiled Newborns.* Clifton, NJ: Humana Press, 1985.

Rothman, D. H. *Strangers at the Bedside.* New York City: Basic Books, 1990 (paperback edition, 1992).

Journals

Cambridge Quarterly of Healthcare Ethics. Published by Cambridge University Press, 40 West 20th Street, New York City, NY 10011.

Hastings Center Report. Published by The Hastings Center, 255 Elm Road, Briarcliff Manor, NY 10510.

HealthCare Ethics Committee (HEC) Forum. Published by Kluwer Academic Publishers, 101 Phillip Drive, Norwell, MA 02061.

The Journal of Clinical Ethics. Published by University Publishing Group, 107 East Church Street, Frederick, MD 21701.

Kennedy Institute of Ethics Journal. Published by Johns Hopkins University Press, Journals Publication Division, 701 W. 40th Street, Suite 275, Baltimore, MD 21211-2190.

Law, Medicine, and Health Care. Published by the American Society of Law, Medicine, and Ethics, 765 Commonwealth Avenue, Boston, MA, 02215.

in determining their content. Other committees do not require course attendance, but strongly recommend it and even allocate funds to pay at least partial tuition costs for some of its members.

Education can include the following:

- *Formal course work:* Usually university based and topic oriented, formal course work may include individual, nonsequential courses, a certificate program of a related series of courses, or a degree program.
- *Informal course work:* Usually facility-based or ethics committee network-based single sessions, informal courses are either topic oriented (for example, a session on euthanasia) or skills oriented (for example, conducting a session on case consults or on evaluating committee work).
- *Internal study groups:* Usually facility based, these typically involve the extended study of a single topic using packets of readings or a single book, and are conducted independently of the ethics committee meeting.
- *Education meetings:* These committee-based meetings typically focus on a single article or case, or involve a didactic presentation.
- *External conferences:* Usually sponsored by organizations outside the facility, these encompass one- and two-day seminars, workshops, symposia, and conferences on both general and specific areas of bioethics.

The ethics committee can provide education through a variety of formats. Films and videotapes; reading materials; and forums for sharing personal experiences, role-playing, conversing, and reflecting are but a few. However, as the following subsections discuss, these formats are often overlooked.

Literature, Film, Personal Experience

Although literature, film, and personal experience are appropriate formats for ethics committee education, committees seldom intentionally use them. This is unfortunate, because typically members easily and deeply relate to these types of formats. For example, we know of no committee that formally spends time reading aloud, discussing short stories about medicine (for example, William Carlos Williams's *Doctor Stories*), watching films (for example, *The Doctor* or Frederick Weissman's *Near Death,* which was broadcast on public television), or allowing members time to discuss their personal experiences in the health care system (although such anecdotal stories often arise spontaneously in the course of committee discussion).

The educational format used by most ethics committees is as restricted as that provided in most academic settings. Were committees to approach education with what Zen calls "the beginner's mind," their efforts might be more effective. According to Zen practitioners, the beginner's mind sees many possibilities; but the more people know, the fewer options they see and, in a sense, the less they know.[2] Having members spend time talking about how they best learn would quickly demonstrate that few do well in a lecture format; yet this is the format most often provided, usually because it is the easiest to provide (despite its relative ineffectiveness in reaching the goal of the education effort).

Role-Playing

Another effective mode of teaching that is seldom used is role-playing. Although many people are self-conscious about role-playing, most participants find it valuable when done frequently in the informal setting of a meeting. Reversing regular roles (having physicians be nurses, chaplains be physicians, nurses be administrators, administrators be family members, and so on) routinely results in people suddenly understanding issues more broadly than they had previously. The most common way to use role-playing is in the mock case review, but it can also be used in other circumstances. For example:

- Have members of the committee go through the hospital admission process or go to clinic appointments in a wheelchair.
- Have members try to do any of the many things that patients/families are expected to do without reading anything (as patients who are not literate or not literate in the dominant language must do).
- Role-play an education session in which the committee tries to explain a new policy to a department that is not sympathetic to it.
- Role-play a meeting with nurses in which they bring ethical issues that trouble them to the attention of the committee.

Role-playing should be followed by a debriefing session in which each person can reflect on what he or she learned. Because the primary reason for this activity is to give people an opportunity to exercise and develop their empathy for others, if they are not given a chance to articulate their feelings about the experience, that experience may not have much effect.

Conversation and Reflection

Most of the educational needs of the committee require opportunities for conversation, reflection, and discussion. Education should help members see how they fit into the world of bioethics and ethics committees. A particularly well-received education session involved a committee member who also belonged to several other ethics committees talking about the differences in ethics committees at different hospitals. Because committees are often isolated in their individual hospitals (and often further isolated within the hospital itself), education that stimulates a sense of being connected to the larger world is important. Having a person who has actually been a surrogate mother talk to the committee about her experience will make for a much more intense and complex discussion of the ethics of surrogate parenting and will connect that discussion to the world outside the hospital. Similarly, having disabled individuals or individuals with chronic illness talk about their experiences with medical care may open the members' minds to more options as they more fully understand what happens when a person becomes a patient and then returns to life outside the hospital.

Videotapes

Videotapes were used for committee education more frequently five years ago than they are today. This is in part because relatively few relevant commercial videotapes are being made, but also because videos are expensive and committee budgets are constrained. Although television frequently covers bioethics issues and some committees make use of this medium, the segments are often too short or too long to be useful. One committee in an urban hospital that had a well-supplied audiovisual department made its own 15-minute video. Using a case that had been particularly troublesome for the committee, the members wrote a script, persuaded hospital staff and physicians to play the roles, and then filmed it themselves. Subsequently, the committee provided copies of the video to other ethics committees in the area. The regional network eventually showed it at a countywide meeting. The success of that video has spurred the committee to work on a second one. Given the increasing availability of video cameras, more committees will likely enter into this area. Committees near universities and colleges with audiovisual departments might want to invite students to join them as colleagues in such endeavors.

Making education creative, involving, and memorable should be the work of ethics committees. Just because they are dealing with ethics does not mean they must be grimly serious in their efforts to educate members.

Responsibility for Committee Education

Responsibility for planning committee education may lie with either the chairperson, a standing subcommittee, a committee member with special expertise in the area, or an outside consultant. One committee simply had each of its members arrange and conduct an educational meeting in his or her respective department during the year on an ethics issue of the member's choice. Although this was an efficient education program, it did not serve to unify the committee in any way because departmental meetings are open only to members of the department, nor did it create any sense of interdisciplinary thinking or working. However, there are other ways to create a sense of community and interdisciplinarity, and this is one means of providing education to the hospital community.

Educational Goals

However education is organized, the committee should establish educational goals. As with treatment goals in medical care, educational goals are easily neglected and educational efforts begin to be carried out for their own sake. Education is at its worst when it becomes only a time slot that must be filled. One committee chairperson announced that, during his tenure, the committee would have a 10-minute education section in each meeting in order to fulfill its education function. Such a formalistic approach is likely to fail (as it did). If the committee does not understand its need for education, it will not make the effort to organize it.

If committees cannot figure out what to do for education, they should contact other ethics committees in their area or contact a regional ethics center or a local ethics committee network (for names and addresses, see appendix 5-1 at the end of the chapter). Sometimes talking with somebody else about the problem provides the kind of jump start that a committee needs to get moving (or to get moving again).

Committees need to determine their own goals relative to their own situation. A 1992 report from a project directed by The Hastings Center on ethics education proposed the following general goals for ethics committees:[3]

- Basic education should be considered in terms of the committee's setting and needs. Ethics committees in long-term care institutions may need to emphasize different issues than those addressed in acute care hospitals; the concerns of ethics committees will differ from those of perinatal committees.
- The scope of the committee's educational efforts must vary depending on the setting and the resources of the committee (both financial and experiential). Availability of speakers, films or videotapes, journals, and special expertise may depend on access to funds and time.
- All education does not come from the ethics committee educational process. Members will increasingly bring with them personal as well as professional knowledge and experience that the committee can use. When members attend conferences and forums, they should be encouraged to share this experience in a manner useful to other committee members.
- The committee's educational program should be assessed from time to time. Do members feel they are learning anything? Are they learning the things they need to know?
- Committees are composed of members with a variety of interests and knowledge levels about bioethics. Additionally, they have new and continuing members. Whether new or continuing, all members are becoming part of a "bioethics conversation" and differing levels of knowledge should be expected. However, anyone invited to this discourse should become sufficiently acquainted with the issues and should attempt to achieve a level 2 understanding. [The Hastings Center report, which deals with bioethics education generally, posits multilevels of achievement, ranging from casual reading to advanced degrees in bioethics.] This includes lay citizens who, for their comfort and the comfort of others, should educate themselves about health care, its language, and its structure.
- Committees that do not have relatively easy access to a bioethics resource person (for example, someone who spends part of his or her working life in the larger field of bioethics) may be at some disadvantage, though sometimes the extraordinary devotion of one or two members who pursued their own education at considerable personal expense accomplishes this function.
- The educational task of an ethics committee is to reach a basic level of knowledge. Committees must continually educate at both basic and ongoing levels with respect to new developments and controversies in the field. Unfortunately, committees often see education as important only during their first year or so and then presume all has been learned.
- Formal education should be as participatory and practical as possible—for example, applied, not theoretical, ethics. "Coverage" of the topic is not the primary goal of these educational sessions; rather, it is whether members can use this information/skill/knowledge in some way.
- Ethics committees should formally devote some time at each meeting to a planned education program.
- Some areas, especially those having little direct impact on the committee, will go unaddressed. Given the limited time available, this is to be expected and is a reasonable establishment of priorities.
- Education of ethics committee members is an ongoing process. After two years on a committee, an individual should feel comfortable in his or her understanding at the basic level of bioethics education. This does not suggest any extraordinary expertise,

however; it is the fundamental information, the information on which intermediate study can be based.

Education outside the Committee

Ethics committees are also expected to provide education for hospital employees, patients and families, and the community at large. Some of the strategies used toward this end are discussed in the remaining subsections.

Educational Approaches

Some committees have been asked by administrators to conduct the education efforts required by the Patient Self-Determination Act on advance directives for staff, physicians, and community members. Some committees have been able to sustain regular (usually monthly) education sessions for health care professionals, either in the form of grand rounds, brown-bag lunches, or noontime lectures. Another approach is "The Ethics Committee Is In." The committee announced a regular day and time when members would be available to anyone in the hospital to discuss patient care issues; it has had a good response. Some committees have been successful with a bioethics week, a yearly event during which the committee sponsors a series of events ranging from lectures and videos to a card table with a notary public available to notarize advance directives for staff and physicians. Other committees have contributed bioethics sessions to organized programs in the institution (for example, during nurse recognition week, committees have presented special sessions on ethical issues of particular importance to nurses; have made presentations at in-service, grand rounds, or orientation programs; or have sponsored joint meetings with institutional review boards). Many have set up multidisciplinary and multiservice meetings on specific topics (such as medicine and psychiatry departments on competency and consent), and worked with case managers and nurse educators to coordinate educational activities and topics. They have obtained the assistance of social workers and psychiatrists in teaching themselves and other members of the hospital community about group process and communication skills.

Educational Topics

Choosing topics for staff education programs may be quite different from determining goals for the committee's self-education. The audience is likely to change from event to event and the number of educational events is likely to be small. Topics should be timely; focusing on cases currently in the news or on issues of particular concern to hospital staff is usually helpful in drawing an audience. Education on new policies can be particularly problematic, because seldom does the perceived need for the policy in the institution match the interest the committee has generated in producing the policy. In the authors' experience, attempting broadscale and direct education on new policies is much less effective than targeting education to small, particularly affected groups. For example, an announcement of the new policy could be conveyed to everyone, but discussions of the policy's details could be directed to those units most likely to be engaged in the activity delineated by the policy.

Educational Tools

Education for staff is also provided in written form. Ethics resource handbooks have been prepared for each nursing unit, with the contents determined by the committee and regularly updated. Some committees have put together traveling resource carts, which include both written materials and videos, particularly intended to help night staff keep up with ethics committee work. Bulletin boards on bioethics in the news are maintained in hospital libraries, physicians' lounges, and corridors. Pamphlets containing summaries of hospital policies with particular bioethical content could be produced and distributed. Members of the Center for

Healthcare Ethics (St. Joseph Health System, Orange, California) receive a quarterly mailing called *Ethical Dimensions,* which they are encouraged to distribute to their staff and physicians. It includes in its general content brief announcements of relevance to the particular hospital. Some committees have regular columns in the institution's newsletter to keep everyone up-to-date on the committee's work. One committee found that its ability to reach out to staff, physicians, and community for education was noticeably improved when a staff member from the hospital's marketing department became a committee member.

As with committee self-education, education for the community will be more effective if it is consistent with the community's perception of its educational needs. Committees that regularly send out surveys and then provide immediate feedback are able to develop a relationship with their communities that makes education interactive: the community needs to participate, not just to be addressed. Surveys beyond needs assessments are very engaging and might focus on topics such as euthanasia, HIV testing for physicians and patients, withholding–withdrawing distinctions, and so on. In getting the results back to the community, it is effective to be able to offer some kinds of comparison — with national numbers, other hospitals, or the same hospital at an earlier date. (See appendix 5-2 for some samples of hospital questionnaires.)

Beyond the hospital confines, committees have worked with local university faculty teaching applied ethics courses to demonstrate case consultation, worked with legislators to develop new legislation and testified before legislative bodies, joined with Health Decision Projects (as in California and Oregon, among others) to provide community education on health care delivery and decision making, written letters to the editor of the local newspaper, participated on radio talk shows, and invited local journalists to report on a program conducted by the ethics committee. Some ethics committees, especially those in more isolated areas, have arranged for regular telephone conference calls with other ethics committees or with someone who has particular expertise in an area of interest. Using speaker phones, committee members are able to share information and to have their questions answered.

Reaching Patients and Families

Many committees have prepared brochures describing hospital policies, medical procedures and the decisions that may need to be made about them (for example, life-sustaining treatment), or the committee's structure and availability to physicians, staff, patients, and families who have ethical concerns about patient care issues. These brochures are often widely distributed and bring the committee some greater degree of recognition. Although considerable effort is often expended in ensuring that the information in the brochure is accurate and complete, seldom is there comparable commitment to ensuring that the brochures are truly accessible to patients.

Educational Level of Written Materials

The language level of educational brochures is often very high and very technical. Typically, ethics committee members are highly educated, both in absolute terms and in comparison with the broader community they serve. They may be very sensitive to these differences in talking to patients, but not in writing to them. One such brochure on CPR talked about "chest compression." When the terminology was challenged as being too technical, the drafter of the text replied: "Well, I can't just say we push down hard on their chest, can I?" The answer should be that if that is the procedure, that is how it should be described. There are inevitable trade-offs among accuracy, delicacy/tactfulness, thoroughness, and comprehensibility in producing such informational brochures. Too often, comprehensibility comes in last.

One way that committees can assess the level of their information is to run it through a simple computer program with a FOG™ index. Such inexpensive programs (one is called FOGFIND™) are available through Shareware™ computer networks. They sample the text and give it a grade-level reading average. (Word for Windows™ 2.0 also has a built-in grammar program that includes several readability indexes.) A second and equally important way is to give the brochure to the kind of people who are its ultimate recipients and ask their opinion about it—about what it says and how it says it. They will be pleased to offer their thoughts and the committee will be in a much better position to judge whether its brochure needs more work. One committee, in developing its forgoing treatment brochure, invited review from approximately 40 laypersons outside the hospital. In addition, members of individual departments—nurse managers, social workers, chaplains, physicians—were personally asked to review and comment. This educated key individuals in the institution and also encouraged a sense of personal involvement in the final product. In a small way, this can lessen the impression that ethical issues are solely the process of the ethics committee.

Translations for Non–English-Speaking Populations

In addition, printed materials are seldom available in the hospital in any language other than English, even in areas of the country where there are substantial numbers of non–English-speaking patients. Obtaining good translations can be a very complex activity and also doubles the printing costs. Part of the problem with obtaining good translations is that the translator may speak and write the language fluently, but not be particularly well informed about the subject of the brochure. Having a second person retranslate the materials back into English is one way for committee members to get some sense of whether the translation communicates what they intended to communicate. The problem of translation in hospitals is greater than that of materials prepared by the ethics committee. Indeed, helping the institution to understand the scope of the problem may be something that ethics committees can take on as a matter of institutional education. Ethics committees might find it helpful to involve someone who is able to provide translation throughout the process of preparing the materials. Ethics committees are notably homogenous in their membership, and ensuring that patients receive important information in a language they speak may be a first step in coming to grips with cultural issues that have largely eluded ethics committees and bioethics generally.

Conclusion

Although case review may be the committee's most noteworthy function, its ability to educate itself and others about the importance and nature of ethical issues in health care will determine its long-term success. Ethics committee members do not own bioethics. However, they are often most interested in the issues and most willing to invest time in learning more about them. Yet, relatively few members choose to read the bioethics literature or attend classes or conferences. It may be that this literature and these conferences have not yet found the way to engage these members, to speak to them in a language that seems helpful. However, the members' presence on the committee and their willingness to attend meetings over time speaks to a genuine interest that has been awakened and is waiting to be engaged.

The initial and first era of ethics committee education has been dominated by philosophical principles/analyses and legal cases. In the future, philosophy and law will continue to be important, but the spotlight may need to move to the values of the institution and of the professionals who work there, as well as to the relationships that do and should exist between them.

Exercises

A. Some questions to ask members about your committee and its education function are:
1. Is there a person on the committee with bioethics background/expertise? Does the committee need one?
2. In planning meetings, does the steering committee consciously address the role of education for all agenda items?
3. Is there a committee to plan education? Would education be more available to more people if there were such a committee?

4. Does the committee chairperson have enough interest in bioethics that he or she would be willing to obtain additional education in the field? Is that necessary?

5. Is there an area network to which chairpersons or committee members can belong? Should there be? Would that make a difference in your committee? Can your committee start such a group?

6. Are there aspects of bioethics with which everybody on the committee ought to be familiar? What are they?

7. Are education needs different in different parts of the institution? For example, does the dialysis unit have different ethical problems than the oncology unit?

B. Sample Test:

1. An advance directive is any spoken or written statement about treatment that a patient wants at some future date.   T   F

2. According to the *Cruzan* case, families cannot refuse artificially supplied nutrition and hydration for permanently unconscious patients.   T   F

3. It is better to withhold treatment from a patient than to withdraw it.   T   F

4. Living wills are recognized by law in this state.   T   F

5. When a patient requests a DNR order, his or her family must be notified before the order is written.   T   F

6. A patient who has an advance directive should have a DNR order written.   T   F

7. This hospital has an institutional review board.   T   F

8. When a patient on a ventilator is found to have irreversibly lost all brain function, including that of the brain stem, the family's consent must be obtained before the ventilator can be turned off.   T   F

9. Patients can give their right to make treatment decisions to someone else, even if they are still mentally able to make their own decisions.   T   F

10. Treatment must always be provided for seriously ill infants, regardless of parental wishes, if the treatment would prolong the infant's life.

C. The "Top 10 Hits" of Bioethics (or Top 30): Six full-time bioethicists were asked to list the 10 most important topics in bioethics from their perspective. This list of 30—in no particular order—is the result of that request. How knowledgeable is your committee about these issues? (For a discussion of these issues, see "References and Notes."[4])

1. *Roe v. Wade*
2. *A.C.* (Cesarean section case)
3. *Johnson Controls* case
4. Karen Quinlan
5. Claire Conroy
6. Nancy Cruzan
7. President's Commission for the Study of Ethical Problems in Medicine and Medical and Biobehavioral Research
8. Kansas Brain Death Statute
9. Harvard Ad Hoc Committee on Irreversible Coma
10. Janet Adkins and Jack Kevorkian
11. *Belmont Report*
12. Oregon Medicaid Priority List
13. Substituted judgment
14. Autonomy–beneficence–justice
15. Education, case consultation, policy development/review
16. Baby Doe, Baby Jane Doe, Baby Doe Regulations and the 1983 amendments to the Child Abuse Law
17. The Hastings Center

18. Dialysis God committees/prognosis committees/ethics committees
19. Dax Cowart and The Texas Burn case
20. *Saikewicz*
21. Elizabeth Bouvia
22. Humane and Dignified Death Act/Initiative
23. Barber–Njedl (The *Herbert* case)
24. Patient Self-Determination Act
25. Henry Beecher and research abuse
26. Asilomar meeting on recombinant DNA
27. Baby Fae
28. Baby M
29. DNR orders and purple dots
30. Advance directives

References and Notes

1. See, for example, Bayley, C. Consultation revisited. *Ethical Currents* 18:3–4, 1989; and Glaser, J. The primary role of ethics committees. *Ethical Currents* 15:3, 8, 1988.

2. Suzuki, S. *Zen Mind, Beginner's Mind.* New York City: Weatherhill, 1970.

3. Thornton, B. C., and Callahan, D. *Bioethics Education: Expanding the Circle.* Briarcliff Manor, NY: The Hastings Center, 1992.

4. Following is a discussion of the issues: *Roe v. Wade*—the 1973 Supreme Court decision making abortion available at least throughout the first two trimesters; *A.C.*—the 1990 Washington, DC, case in which a cesarean section was performed over the objection of the pregnant woman (who was terminally ill and expected to die soon) and her parents, on the grounds that the fetus might be viable (the infant died), but the appellate court held that the wishes of the pregnant woman should be determinative in such situations, except in very unusual circumstances; *Johnson Controls*—the 1990 U.S. Supreme Court case in which it was argued that women could not be discriminated against in the workplace on the grounds that they might become pregnant; Karen Quinlan—the subject of a 1976 New Jersey Supreme Court case that closed the first era of bioethics or opened the second one by announcing that Ms. Quinlan's right of privacy could be exercised by her father with respect to stopping the respirator if it were found that she would never return to a "cognitive and sapient state"; Claire Conroy—the subject of a 1985 New Jersey Supreme Court case, the first in which it was concluded that artificially supplied food and fluid could be forgone for patients under specific circumstances; Nancy Cruzan—the subject of a 1991 U.S. Supreme Court case, the first in which the highest court held that a state was entitled to establish standards of proof about a patient's wishes with respect to receiving or forgoing treatment; President's Commission—the second national commission on bioethics and the author of 11 volumes of reports on treatment decisions and access issues; Kansas Brain Death Statute—the first state law (1970) to define death in terms of whole brain criteria as well as cardiorespiratory function; Harvard Ad Hoc Committee on Irreversible Coma—the committee that published standards for diagnosing whole brain death in 1968, although confusing the issue by calling it irreversible coma; Janet Adkins and Dr. Jack Kevorkian—the patient diagnosed with Alzheimer's disease who wanted a lethal injection and the Michigan pathologist who wanted to provide it for her (the 1991 case that galvanized the public on the issue of legalizing active euthanasia); *Belmont Report*—the 1979 seminal report by the first national commission on bioethics that exclusively addressed issues of ethics and use of human subjects in research (the report articulated the central principles of patient autonomy, beneficence, and justice as the relevant values to be analyzed in establishing public policy in this area); Oregon Medicaid Priority List—the first formal attempt to ration health care to a discrete population on the basis of cost-effectiveness; substituted judgment—the decision-making standard that presumed those closest to the patient could use their knowledge of the patient to judge what the patient would actually want if he or she were currently able to convey a preference, a claim that has not been demonstrated through subsequent empirical research; autonomy–beneficence–justice—the "Georgetown Mantra" and the principles conceded to govern treatment decisions; education, case consultation, policy development/review—the three functions of ethics committees; Baby Doe, Baby Jane Doe, Baby Doe Regulations, and the 1983 amendments to the Child Abuse Law—two cases and two sets of regulations that engaged the

public and professionals on the issue of what treatment should be provided for seriously ill disabled newborns and whether their parents should be allowed to decide that treatment was not to be provided; The Hastings Center—the best-known and among the oldest of the bioethics research centers and the publisher of the *Hastings Center Report,* the best known of the bioethics journals; dialysis God committees, prognosis committees, and ethics committees—the historical lineage of the ethics committee; dialysis God committees chose patients in Seattle to receive dialysis when there were more patients than equipment, the prognosis committees were to ensure that patients for whom treatment was to be forgone (as in the case of Karen Quinlan) would not return to a sapient and cognitive state; Dax Cowart and the Texas Burn Case—a young man seriously burned in a gas explosion in 1973 who refused treatment but was treated anyway, who had two films made about his case, and who became a national spokesperson for patients' rights to refuse treatment; *Saikewicz*—a 1977 Massachusetts case in which a decision was made to withhold chemotherapy from a seriously retarded man with cancer; Elizabeth Bouvia—a California quadriplegic who in her second case (1986) successfully argued that she was entitled to refuse forced feeding, even if she were not terminally ill; Humane and Dignified Death Act/Initiative—the initiative conducted in Washington in 1991 (and in California in 1992) to permit physicians to provide lethal injections for terminally ill patients who request such assistance; Barber–Njedl (the *Herbert* case)—a 1983 California case in which two physicians had criminal homicide charges filed against them for withdrawing a feeding tube from a patient believed to be irreversibly comatose (the charges were subsequently dropped); Patient Self-Determination Act—the 1990 federal law requiring health care institutions that receive Medicare or Medicaid funds to inform patients/clients/residents/members about their rights to refuse or consent to treatment and to make advance directives under their state law; Henry Beecher and research abuse—the distinguished Harvard physician and faculty member who wrote in 1966 about the extent to which human subjects were unethically used in research, usually without their knowledge or without their knowledge of the harm they risked, which led to the establishment of the first federal commission on ethics in medicine in 1974; Asilomar meeting on recombinant DNA—the 1972 meeting called by scientists involved in research on recombinant DNA (and attended almost exclusively by such scientists) whose agenda was to explore safety issues and to ensure to the greatest degree possible self-regulation in this area of research; Baby Fae—the infant who, in 1985, was given a baboon's heart in a transplant effort that ultimately failed; Baby M—the child born in 1987 in a surrogacy arrangement and whose genetic mother ultimately refused to give the child to the contracting parents, which led to a custody case in which the genetic mother lost custody but retained visiting rights; DNR orders and purple dots—the situation reported in 1984 that arose in a New York hospital in which DNR orders were not recorded, but purple dot labels were placed on file cards identifying which patients were not to be resuscitated (the problem with the method gained public attention when a patient was not resuscitated and some cards were found to have more than one purple dot, suggesting that dots were slipping onto other cards); advance directives—written documents in which individuals specify either whom they want to make treatment decisions for them or how they want treatment decisions made should they lose the capacity to make their own decisions.

Appendix 5-1. Bioethics Networks and Centers

Bioethics centers, programs, networks, and institutes are springing up throughout the country and a complete listing of all such groups would be very lengthy. Those listed below are ones that the authors know to have some particular interest in ethics committees and should serve as resources for individuals in different regions of the country.

West Coast

Alice Vrolyk Bioethics Institute
Northridge Hospital Medical Center
18300 Roscoe Boulevard
Northridge, CA 91328

Center for Biomedical Ethics
Stanford University
701B Welch Road, Suite 222
Palo Alto, CA 94305

Center for Christian Ethics
Loma Linda University
Loma Linda, CA 92350

Center for Healthcare Ethics
and Orange County Bioethics Network
St. Joseph Health System
440 S. Batavia Street
Orange, CA 92668

International Bioethics Institute
1721 Mar West
Tiburon, CA 94920

Los Angeles County Ethics Committee Network
c/o David Blake, Department of Philosophy
Loyola Marymount University
Los Angeles, CA 90045

Pacific Center for Health Policy and Ethics
University of Southern California Law Center
Los Angeles, CA 90089-0071

Pacific Northwest

Center for Ethics in Health Care
and Health Ethics Network of Oregon
Oregon Health Sciences University
3181 S.W. Sam Jackson Park Road, L101
Portland, OR 97201

Northwest Network of Ethics Committees
310 Tacoma Avenue
Tacoma, WA 98403

Rocky Mountains

Division of Medical Ethics
LDS Hospital and University of Utah
8th Avenue and C Street
Salt Lake City, UT 84143

The Institute of Medicine and Humanities
St. Patrick Hospital and University of Montana
P.O. Box 4587
Missoula, MT 59812

Southwest

Center for Health Law and Ethics
Institute of Public Law
University of New Mexico
Albuquerque, NM 87131

Program in Bioethics
University of Arizona College of Medicine
Tucson, AZ 85724

Midwest

Center for Biomedical Ethics
Case Western Reserve University School of Medicine
10900 Euclid Avenue
Cleveland, OH 44106

Center for Health Care Ethics
St. Louis University Medical Center
1402 S. Grand Boulevard
St. Louis, MO 63104

Department of Bioethics, P-31
Cleveland Clinic Foundation
9500 Euclid Avenue
Cleveland, OH 44195

Department of Medical Jurisprudence and Humanities
University of Nebraska Medical Center
600 S. 42nd Street
Omaha, NE 68198

Medical Humanities Program
Loyola Stritch School of Medicine
2160 S. First Avenue
Maywood, IL 60153

Michigan Ethics Resource Network
c/o The Center for Ethics and Humanities in the Life Sciences
C-201 East Fee Hall
Michigan State University
East Lansing, MI 48824-1316

Midwest Bioethics Center
410 Archibald, Suite 200
Kansas City, MO 64111-3000

Minnesota Network for Institutional Ethics Committees
c/o Minnesota Hospital Association
2221 University Avenue, SE, Suite 425
Minneapolis, MN 55414-3085

North Dakota Institutional Ethics Committee Network
c/o Division of Ethics and Humanities
University of North Dakota School of Medicine
501 N. Columbia Road
Grand Forks, ND 58201

The Park Ridge Center
211 E. Ontario, Suite 800
Chicago, IL 60611

Wisconsin Ethics Committee Network
c/o Center for the Study of Bioethics
Medical College of Wisconsin
8701 Watertown Plank Road
Milwaukee, WI 53226

Northeast

Division of Humanities in Medicine
State University of New York
Health Science Center at Brooklyn
450 Clarkson Avenue
Brooklyn, NY 11203

The Hastings Center
255 Elm Road
Briarcliff Manor, NY 10510

Vermont Ethics Network
103 S. Main Street
Waterbury, VT 05671-1401

Atlantic Seaboard

Center for Medical Ethics
University of Pittsburgh
3400 Forbes Avenue, Suite 506
Pittsburgh, PA 15213

Florida Bioethics Network
c/o Medical Humanities Program, J-222
College of Medicine
Gainesville, FL 32610

Maryland Institutional Ethics Committee Resource Network
Law and Health Care Program
University of Maryland School of Law
500 W. Baltimore Street
Baltimore, MD 21202-1786

South

Center for Biomedical Ethics
Health Sciences Center
University of Virginia, P.O. Box 348
Charlottesville, VA 22908

Department of Human Values and Ethics
University of Tennessee—Memphis
956 Court Street, P.O. Box 11
Memphis, TN 38163

Department of Medical Humanities
School of Medicine
East Carolina University
Greenville, NC 27858

Kennedy Institute of Ethics
Georgetown University
Poulton Hall
37th and P Streets
Washington, DC 20057

Appendix 5-2. Samples of Hospital Questionnaires

Our Ethics Committee Needs Your Help!

_____ Hospital Ethics Committee is conducting a survey to assess current awareness of and need for information and education in bioethics. Please take a moment to complete this survey.

1. Are you aware that we have an Ethics Committee?   ___ Yes ___ No

2. Our committee is planning educational programs for the coming year. Please check _only three (3) topics_ you are most interested in:

   ___ Principles of ethical decision making
   ___ DNR guidelines
   ___ Allocation of resources
   ___ Informed consent
   ___ Pain management
   ___ Providing different levels of care for patients with different means of payment
   ___ Providing treatments that are medically futile
   ___ Withholding or withdrawing artificial nutrition/hydration

   ___ Determining a patient's competence
   ___ Confidentiality
   ___ Ethical issues in AIDS
   ___ Physician-assisted suicide/euthanasia
   ___ Communication difficulties among staff
   ___ Deciding when to consider the economic implications of a patient's care
   ___ Dealing with noncompliant patients
   ___ Durable power of attorney and other advance directives

3. Please indicate your position:
   ___ Medical staff
   ___ Ancillary, patient care
   ___ Other _____

   ___ Nursing
   ___ Administration

   ___ Social work
   ___ Support services

4. Would you be interested in being a member of the Ethics Committee if an opening becomes available? (If yes, please sign this form)   ___ Yes ___ No

Signature (optional): _____

AIDS

1. Our institution has dealt well with most aspects concerning AIDS.

___ strongly agree   ___ agree   ___ not sure   ___ disagree   ___ strongly disagree

Comments:

2. I feel well informed about who is responsible for handling AIDS issues and what has been done in this regard.

___ strongly agree   ___ agree   ___ not sure   ___ disagree   ___ strongly disagree

Comments:

3. I believe that our ethics committee is well informed about the major ethical aspects of AIDS.

___ strongly agree   ___ agree   ___ not sure   ___ disagree   ___ strongly disagree

Comments:

4. I believe that our employees are well informed about the major aspects of AIDS.

___ strongly agree   ___ agree   ___ not sure   ___ disagree   ___ strongly disagree

Comments:

5. I believe that our patients/families are well informed about the major aspects of AIDS.

___ strongly agree   ___ agree   ___ not sure   ___ disagree   ___ strongly disagree

Comments:

6. I believe that we have adequate policies and practices concerning AIDS for

Medical staff:

___ strongly agree   ___ agree   ___ not sure   ___ disagree   ___ strongly disagree

Comments:

Employees:

___ strongly agree   ___ agree   ___ not sure   ___ disagree   ___ strongly disagree

Comments:

Patients:

___ strongly agree   ___ agree   ___ not sure   ___ disagree   ___ strongly disagree

Comments:

7. List as many things as you can think of that the ethics committee could do to improve the present situation.

8. Of all the items you listed in number 7, which two deserve priority attention?

Questionnaire for Physicians on Advance Directives

1. How familiar are you with advance directives for health care?

   ___ very familiar   ___ somewhat familiar   ___ barely familiar   ___ totally ignorant

2. Have you completed some form of advance directive?

   ___ yes   ___ no

3. Do you intend to complete some form of advance directive?

   ___ yes   ___ no

4. Have members of your family completed some form of advance directive?

   ___ yes   ___ no

5. What percentage of your colleagues do you think have completed some form of advance directive?

   ___ 5% or less   ___ 10%   ___ 20%   ___ 30%   ___ 40%

6. What percentage of your patients do you think have completed some form of advance directive?

   ___ 5% or less   ___ 10%   ___ 20%   ___ 30%   ___ 40%

7. I believe that advance directives have very limited usefulness.

   ___ strongly agree   ___ agree   ___ not sure   ___ disagree   ___ strongly disagree

8. How many situations do you know of where an advance directive would have helped resolve a difficulty?

   ___ quite a few   ___ some   ___ hardly any   ___ none

9. What percentage of your patients have mentioned advance directives to you?

   ___ 5% or less   ___ 10%   ___ 20%   ___ 30%   ___ 40%

10. I would like to discuss advance directives with my patients.

    ___ strongly agree   ___ agree   ___ not sure   ___ disagree   ___ strongly disagree

11. I plan to discuss advance directives with my patients.

    ___ strongly agree   ___ agree   ___ not sure   ___ disagree   ___ strongly disagree

12. I think that discussing advance directives with my patients would not be a good use of my clinical time.

    ___ strongly agree   ___ agree   ___ not sure   ___ disagree   ___ strongly disagree

Questionnaire for Physicians on Anencephalic Infants

1. I believe that anencephalic infants should be treated with the same care as any other seriously ill child.

   ___ strongly agree ___ agree ___ not sure ___ disagree ___ strongly disagree

   Comment:

2. I believe that anencephalic infants are substantially different from other infants.

   ___ strongly agree ___ agree ___ not sure ___ disagree ___ strongly disagree

   Comment:

3. I believe that it is ethically acceptable to harvest the organs of anencephalic infants even before they are brain dead.

   ___ strongly agree ___ agree ___ not sure ___ disagree ___ strongly disagree

   Comment:

4. I believe that the condition of anencephaly is ethically the equivalent of brain death.

   ___ strongly agree ___ agree ___ not sure ___ disagree ___ strongly disagree

   Comment:

5. I believe that the condition of anencephaly is legally the equivalent of brain death.

   ___ strongly agree ___ agree ___ not sure ___ disagree ___ strongly disagree

   Comment:

6. I believe that we should—as they now do in Germany—make it public policy that parents can consent to donate the organs of their anencephalic infant even though he/she is not brain dead.

   ___ strongly agree ___ agree ___ not sure ___ disagree ___ strongly disagree

   Comment:

General Questionnaire

1. Eventually we should change the definition of *brain death* from whole brain death to neocortical death.

   ___ strongly agree   ___ agree   ___ not sure   ___ disagree   ___ strongly disagree

2. Some demented states are so severe that they are equivalent to persistent vegetative state in making ethical decisions.

   ___ strongly agree   ___ agree   ___ not sure   ___ disagree   ___ strongly disagree

3. Caring for patients in PVS can be a source of ethical conflict for caregivers.

   ___ strongly agree   ___ agree   ___ not sure   ___ disagree   ___ strongly disagree

4. I want the financial cost to the community to be a factor in my surrogate's decision about my care when I am no longer able to decide.

   ___ strongly agree   ___ agree   ___ not sure   ___ disagree   ___ strongly disagree

5. Concerning the condition of persistent vegetative state —

   For myself, I would consider that:

   ___ better than being dead   ___ equivalent to being dead   ___ worse than being dead

   Society should treat this condition as:

   ___ better than being dead   ___ equivalent to being dead   ___ worse than being dead
   ___ not society's judgment to make

   I believe that medical treatment for a person in that state should be limited:

   ___ severely   ___ somewhat   ___ not at all   ___not my judgment to make

6. Concerning an irreversible condition with only dim and intermittent recognition of others—

   For myself, I would consider that:

   ___ better than being dead   ___ equivalent to being dead   ___ worse than being dead

   Society should treat this condition as:

   ___ better than being dead   ___ equivalent to being dead   ___ worse than being dead
   ___ not society's judgment to make

   I believe that medical tx for a person in that state should be limited:

   ___ severely   ___ somewhat   ___ not at all   ___not my judgment to make

7. Concerning an irreversible condition where one is conscious but has totally lost continuity with his or her past—

   For myself, I would consider that:

   ___ better than being dead   ___ equivalent to being dead   ___ worse than being dead

   Society should treat this condition as:

   ___ better than being dead   ___ equivalent to being dead   ___ worse than being dead
   ___ not society's judgment to make

   I believe that medical treatment for a person in that state should be limited:

   ___ severely   ___ somewhat   ___ not at all   ___not my judgment to make

Source: Center for Healthcare Ethics, a service of St. Joseph Health System, Orange, CA.

6

Policies and Guidelines: When They Should Be Written

There is relatively little in the ethics committee literature on policy and guideline writing, even though this activity is a staple for most committees.[1] Indeed, the very fact that so little information on policy and guideline writing is available in the literature seems to suggest it is an appropriate activity for committees to undertake. However, the reasons for performing this activity need to be thought out and seriously considered; otherwise, committees are likely to find themselves writing policies because others need them and not because they think the policies are important. If that begins to happen, their policy and guideline writing activity could become just another bureaucratic function in the institution.

Which should committees write, policies or guidelines? Initially, they were more inclined to write guidelines, probably because committees were unsure of their authority and their acceptance in the institution and guidelines were likely to be less threatening to their colleagues. Now, at least in some parts of the country, ethics committees are writing policy, particularly on forgoing treatment. To some extent, this is happening because committees are more secure about their authority and status in the institution. More important, however, is the emergence of a strong national consensus on the appropriate ethical stand to be reflected in forgoing life-sustaining treatment policies. Thus, in writing local policy, individual committees can cite a number of external authorities (for example, The President's Commission,[2] The Hastings Center,[3] The Appleton consensus document,[4] professional medical codes,[5] and various court cases[6]) as justification for their recommendations. As a result, a committee proposal will not be perceived as simply the opinion of a single group of people in one particular hospital.

Thus, much of the policy and guideline writing that has taken place in the past five years has been a matter of catching up with the well-documented consensus in well-delineated areas: definitions of death, DNR orders, forgoing life-sustaining treatment (such as ventilators and dialysis), forgoing artificially supplied nutrition and hydration, and use of advance directives.

However, some committees are also branching out into areas where there is no clear consensus and often the law is unclear (for example, withholding/withdrawing "futile" treatment, making treatment decisions for incapacitated patients who have no one to serve as a surrogate, testing source patients for HIV infection without consent when they are unable to give consent,[7] and relating treatment decisions to resource allocation [for example, ICU admission and discharge guidelines[8]]). On such topics, the committee is likely to return to writing guidelines, less because committee members fear exceeding their authority within the institution, than because a broad national consensus has not yet developed. The remainder of this chapter uses the term *policy* as a general designation, with the understanding that committees should make their own determination as to whether they wish to recommend a policy or guidelines in specific instances.

The Purpose of Institutional Policy

For some, the primary purpose of institutional policy is to provide legal protection and their only concern is whether it conforms to whatever the law permits. This is a narrow view of policy, although it is one that must be acknowledged. Administrators (and many clinicians as well) often view policies as essential statements of rules: if X happens, do Y. Although this is somewhat broader than the legal protection view, it misses the mark by assuming that the complex situations regularly occurring in patient care can be captured in simple rule statements. This conception also tends to suggest that if the policy does not specifically say you can do something, you cannot do it. In bioethics, policies are more likely to be understood, at least in part, as a description of how to think a complex problem through rather than simply as what to do when the bottom line is reached.

Ethics committees would be well advised to think of policy as one way in which the institution can translate the abstract values of its mission statement into practical terms. It is easy to say that the institution is committed to treating people fairly, but how does the institution plan to do that in the case of patients with inadequate insurance? It is easy to say that patients will be treated with respect, but how will that respect be shown when they refuse treatment that caregivers believe to be necessary for them or request treatment that caregivers believe to be inappropriate? If hospitals and medical centers are to be taken seriously as moral communities, they must create policies that deal with the difficult questions as well as the easy ones. Waiting until someone else achieves consensus means waiting until someone else defines the institution's moral values.

If the purpose of policy is to demonstrate institutional values, the committee must be clear about what those values are. In religion-based hospitals, for example, staff and physicians often are not members of the religious community that operates the hospital. Nevertheless, they must understand the central values of that religion and the way in which those values affect the provision of health care. In public hospitals, mission statements are less specific and there is often ambiguity (and perhaps ambivalence) about whether justice or beneficence is the central value. For example, should the poor who are the primary recipients of treatment in county hospitals be treated fairly or kindly? (Obviously both, if both are possible; but sometimes these values conflict. Refusing to make repeated allowances for the indigent patient with renal failure who does not live up to a negotiated treatment contract would be fair, but it might not be kind. A decision to replace, several times, heart valves that become infected as a result of IV drug use takes scarce resources away from other patients. Doing so may be kind, but it may not be fair.)

Teaching hospitals, health maintenance organizations (HMOs), community not-for-profit hospitals, and private for-profit hospitals may understand their missions differently, leading to subtle but distinct differences in their moral stance. For example, special patient suites with abundant amenities may make perfect sense in terms of the values of the for-profit hospital but not those of the HMO. Increasing patient access to research protocols may be more appropriate in the teaching hospital than in the community hospital. Committees should spend some time, even if they have been in existence for a while, elucidating their institution's primary values and considering whether the institution's practices actually reflect those values. (Such a discussion might, for example, make clear that the institution's official values are a commitment to providing accessible health care for members of the community, whereas its actual practices involve excluding many members of the community either because the institution is not sensitive to language or cultural differences or because it does not value them particularly.)

Unless ethics committees are willing to help the institution become more specific about what affirming its values means—about which everybody is enthusiastic in their general form—health care as a moral enterprise makes no headway. Justice, for example, has to do with treatment decisions, as well as with criteria for leadership. Not all issues that deal with justice are matters for the ethics committee. However, it is the ethics committee's task to observe where practices, policies, and mission have become disconnected and to at least suggest to some other group in the institution that the issue be pursued.

The Patient Self-Determination Act (PSDA) requires that health care institutions tell their patients/clients in advance about their policies with respect to state laws on consent to and refusal of treatment and execution of advance directives. This may be a first step in expecting hospitals to tell patients about their values. As they are urged to find physicians who share their values, in the future patients are likely to be urged to find a hospital that shares their values. It is worth noting that in several judicial decisions involving health care institutions that were unwilling to stop treatment, the court required that the institution have in place, in advance, a policy stating that it would not carry out certain actions and that the patient needed to be informed of this at admission.

If institutions expect to act on their values, they need to be clear about their values and about how those values will be realized in their actions. Institutional policies are the locus of information about this realization. It is in this context that ethics committees are expected to have some special role in policy writing and recommendation.

When the Committee Writes a Policy

Generally, policies should be created only when there is a widespread and repeated problem, a pattern of actions that are inconsistent with the institution's values. Even then, there should be a period of questioning whether the problem is best addressed by a policy, education, or both. Education, improved communication, and attention to structures that distribute power ineffectively or inappropriately all may be better ways of addressing the problem than with a policy. Hospitals probably already have too many policies, the large majority of which are unknown to physicians and staff and often are inconsistent with facility practices. Policy writing works best when it is seen as part of a larger educational effort.

Should Policy Be Written When the Administration Needs a Policy?

Several years ago, when the Joint Commission on Accreditation of Healthcare Organizations (JCAHO) issued a requirement that hospitals have written DNR policies, many hospital administrators interpreted this to mean that the hospital was required to have an ethics committee in order to write DNR policies. This is notable because it demonstrates how closely ethics committees and policy writing have been linked. It is also notable because it demonstrates how ethics committees can be undermined from the beginning if they are treated as ad hoc committees formed to complete specific tasks. There is certainly nothing wrong (either ethically or administratively) in creating an ad hoc committee to write a DNR policy for the facility if one is required, but the committee should not be called an ethics committee.

Having an externally delegated task as the formative process for an ethics committee is almost certain to lead to an ethics committee without cohesion. It would be better to create an ad hoc group to write the policy and another group to become an ethics committee, whose immediate tasks are to determine what the institution needs from an ethics committee and possibly to review the policy written by the ad hoc group. An existing ethics committee may take on assigned policy-writing tasks from administration, but the committee should be clear about why it has been asked to do so. Is it because the committee is knowledgeable about the subject? Is the administration asking the committee to judge how the facility should respond to specific situations? Or, is the committee's purpose simply to codify what the administration has already concluded? If it is the latter, it is difficult to see why this is an ethics committee task.

Should Policy Be Written in Response to the Ethics Literature?

As the literature fills with articles on forgoing futile treatment, some ethics committees have considered incorporating the futility concept into their own policies on DNR or forgoing life-sustaining treatment. Although this can be a very useful educational exercise, writing a policy because an issue is being discussed by others is likely to generate a policy that has little effect. Thus, the policy is likely to be written, filed, and forgotten. However, the process of exploring such a topic may provide the committee with a much better understanding of the issues and, in time, may lead to a more internally motivated desire for such a policy. It may be that the issue is perceived in the hospital, but not in the terms that are being discussed in the literature, and that a discussion will reformulate the perception and the sense of institutional need. It may also lead to a decision not to pursue such a policy. For example, one committee explored revising its DNR policy with respect to futile requests for resuscitation and concluded that it could not write a policy stating that CPR would be denied to a competent patient who wanted it, even when the treatment team unanimously agreed that CPR would be futile. Although no policy revision was issued, the committee understood that it had not wasted its time in the process but, rather, had advanced its own understanding of the issue and its own values.

Should Policy Be Written in Response to a Difficult Case?

In law, it is said that hard cases make bad law. Likewise, hard medical cases probably make bad hospital policy. It is tempting to think that a policy would make a hard case easier to resolve, but probably it would not. No number of ethics committees or ethics committee policies will eliminate the hard cases. If the same hard case shows up repeatedly, it may be time to consider a policy, though the policy may be addressed not at resolving the hard case but at interventions to keep it from becoming a hard case. For example, at one hospital conflicts between families and long-time companions of individuals with AIDS led not to a policy on which one should be the decision maker but, rather, to a policy on giving patients diagnosed with AIDS fast-track access to advance directive information. (This was prior to the PSDA requirements.) Similarly, hard cases of families who want extensive treatment for patients in a persistent vegetative state (PVS) may best be addressed by policies that require regular case conferences when a diagnosis of PVS is considered or that require involvement of consultation–liaison psychiatry or social work with family members, rather than by policies that deal with futile treatment.

Should Policy Be Written When There Is a Clear Institutional Need?

Ethics committees ought to consider writing policy when a substantial minority of its members conclude that an area of institutional practice affecting the organization's values is subject to so much discretion that professionals (nurses, physicians, or others) are too frequently being forced to act against their values and/or patients are too frequently being treated against their values. *Too frequently* is obviously a vague standard, but if those who are asked by the institution to act as ethical security guards find it too frequent, that should be acceptable as the point at which the issue needs to be addressed.

In many institutions, committees write a policy only when it is suggested by someone else. It is not uncommon for committees to spend long periods of time on a policy they believe should exist (for example, DNR), even though it is not their greatest area of practical concern or what they care most about. For example, one committee assigned its policy group to work on futility issues, even though the committee members' greater concern was pain control.

A more positive approach would be for committees to occasionally conduct needs assessments of their members or of their institution's staff and physicians to determine what areas of practice could benefit from new policies (or from clearer or more specific policies). Helping people solve real problems is more rewarding than helping to solve theoretical or paper problems. Policy writing should be motivated by real practice needs and backed by professionals', patients', and committee members' emotional commitment to the need.

The Policies That Committees Write

Policies written by institutional ethics committees cluster largely around forgoing treatment issues. A recent survey of Catholic hospitals in California found that they seldom had holistic forgoing treatment policies; in other words, they were not likely to have a single policy addressing forgoing treatment. Instead, they were more likely to have one policy on forgoing resuscitation, one on forgoing artificially supplied nutrition and hydration, one on forgoing life-sustaining treatment, and one on advance directives. This probably resulted not from a decision to create separate policies but from the fact that the topics "matured" at different times and thus were addressed independently. A noticeable downside to these separated policies is that they often lacked consistency, in both form and substance. One policy might have definitions of terms, and another might not. Even those with defined terms often would not define them in the same way. Similarly, principles were defined differently or different principles were introduced as the basis for similar decisions. For example, in one policy *justice* appeared as a principle justifying forgoing artificially supplied nutrition and hydration, but not as one justifying forgoing resuscitation.

It is time that committees having such separate policies combine them into a single forgoing life-sustaining treatment policy (or even a life-sustaining treatment decision policy). It would be appropriate to include subsections to highlight special circumstances (for example, DNR orders that represent an unusual case of consent required for *not* performing a procedure). The argument against such a comprehensive policy is that it may be too long to be helpful. One way to address this problem would be to write a single policy that is introduced by an abbreviated version, with references to the larger policy so that users could find the issues about which they needed to know more. Indeed, given the frequent claim that policy is known only to the policy writers, a comprehensive policy with a good index might be suitable for a short brochure that could then be used as the basis for comprehensive education in the facility. Just as patients would receive brochures providing uniform information on their rights to consent to or refuse treatment and to make advance directives (under the Patient Self-Determination Act), new employees and staff physicians could be given information on the facility's ethical standards for providing health care.

Following is a list of topics for which ethics committees have written policies (gleaned from both the authors' experience and the available literature):

- Advance directive information and use
- Brain death
- Confidentiality
- Consent for HIV testing
- Determining appropriate surrogates for patients who lack capacity for decision making
- Determining patients' capacity for decision making
- DNR orders
- DNR orders in surgery
- Donation of anencephalic newborns' organs by parents
- Use of expensive and minimally effective drugs (for example, thromboplastin activator [TPA])
- Forgoing artificially supplied nutrition and hydration
- Forgoing life-sustaining treatment
- Informed consent
- Interinstitutional transfer orders
- In vitro fertilization patient selection
- Life-sustaining treatment decisions
- Maternal–fetal conflicts
- Surrogate motherhood and consent
- Pain relief administration
- Refusal of blood transfusion by Jehovah's Witnesses
- Sterilization
- Treatment decisions for seriously ill newborns
- Treatment for rape victims

There do not appear to be separate policies exclusively addressing either futile treatment (although a number of committees have written policies that incorporate concern with futile treatment into both DNR and forgoing treatment policies) or CPR (as opposed to DNR). Various sample policies, including two forgoing treatment policies that address the futility issue and a CPR policy are presented in appendix 6-1. The CPR policy clearly addresses some aspects of the futile resuscitation problem, as well as physicians' unwillingness to discuss resuscitation with patients or their families.

Several years ago, there was some enthusiasm for trying to change the concept of DNR orders so that an order would be required for CPR (the patient would not be resuscitated in the event of a cardiorespiratory arrest unless a CPR order had been written). No facility appears to have attempted this policy change, although some have reported changing the wording of the current order from "do-not-resuscitate" to "do-not-attempt resuscitation," in an attempt to clarify to patients and their families that resuscitation is not guaranteed by the resuscitation effort. This is an important linguistic difference and one that ethics committees might consider.

Because choice of language is often not taken very seriously in health care, effecting such a change might be difficult. However, miscommunications and misperceptions (as well as problematic requests for CPR) might thereby be averted. It is one thing to ask the family to consent to *not resuscitating* a patient and quite another to ask them to consent to *not attempting resuscitation,* with the clear implication that the procedure would not be successful.

Different Approaches to Policy Writing

There is wide variation in how committees approach policy writing. Some involve the whole group, others have standing committees for this purpose, and still others create ad hoc committees to write a particular policy. Still other committees see policy writing as part of an educational effort or as part of their policy review function. In the final analysis, the approach chosen by the ethics committee must be one that fits its culture.

Whole Committee Approach

Often, small and fairly new committees write policy as a group. This means that most or all of the time of committee meetings is spent debating policy content and how it is to be phrased. It also usually means that the committee spends many months without completing the policy. Some committees seem to thrive on this process, others seem to be totally dispirited by it.

The members of a committee who work together to produce an important policy are all likely to understand its nuances thoroughly, to be able to explain and defend their choices, and to help others understand the policy more effectively than are members of committees who do not work in this way. However, they are also likely to spend a great deal of limited committee time arguing about issues that are primarily procedural rather than ethical, for example, whether a DNR order should be reviewed every 36, 48, or 72 hours. Having policy writing dominate the whole committee in this way may be good if the members are comfortable with one another (because much of their time will be spent arguing about what to put in the policy and how to phrase it). If the committee has retained the hospital's hierarchical style or if a few members dominate the committee, the experience will be frustrating or discouraging for members who either are not participating or do not feel invited to participate in the discussion.

Although this approach can be very stimulating—a kind of intellectual free-for-all—its success depends on the committee's deeper structure and its willingness to wait a long time for a final result. We have seen committees successfully adopt this style and work on a policy revision for a year or more. Clearly, they perceive the process primarily as an educational activity whose secondary goal is the actual policy.

Standing Subcommittees

Other committees have a standing subcommittee whose sole task is to determine which policies the ethics committee needs to write, and to draft and revise policies for the whole committee's approval. Members usually volunteer to participate on the subcommittee, which means that they are more likely to have an interest in this function. The strength of this method is that the drafting and much of the detail work take place offstage, as it were, rather than during regular ethics committee meetings. Furthermore, this method lets subcommittee members establish a kind of ownership over their work, which they may find very rewarding. Usually, policies created this way are completed more rapidly—sometimes within a few months—because the whole committee needs only address the central issues.

However, one drawback is that the whole committee may not clearly understand the central issues. During the process of completing the policy draft, the subcommittee makes many choices, some of an important ethical nature. The whole committee may not understand either where those choices were made or their implications. The subcommittee should keep track of where the thorny areas are (or were) and report on them when discussing the draft with the full committee.

Often, the subcommittee goes through exhausting discussion of a single point and, having finally reached some consensus, becomes understandably invested in that consensus and assumes that it speaks for the whole committee. For example, after extensive debate one subcommittee decided to specify in the policy that no decision to forgo nutrition and hydration could be based on financial concerns unless they were the patient's own concerns. The whole committee, however, saw the issue differently, which led to considerable negotiation between the whole committee and the subcommittee about how the final draft should address this issue. (The final policy stated that if financial concerns were any part of the basis of the decision, that fact should be documented.)

Ad Hoc Committees

Some committees appoint an ad hoc committee to work on a policy when there is a need for policy writing. The advantage to this approach is that those who are particularly interested in that policy are likely to participate (which is not necessarily true of standing subcommittees on policy). On the other hand, some committees have a handful of people who do all the work; ad hoc committees often comprise those same few people.

Policy Writing as Education

Committees occasionally use policy writing as a stimulus to think about a topic on which there is little consensus. For example, one committee chairperson drafted a policy stating that at the hospital in question, resuscitative efforts would never be made for infants who weighed less than 500 grams. The chairperson presented it to the committee as a way of getting members to think about whether and how such a policy would support or vary from the institution's values and the community's expectations. Such an effort, whether about very small newborns, surrogate mothers, or ICU admission/discharge criteria, might ultimately become the basis for a new policy if it were able to capture a view that fit the hospital's values.

Policy Writing as Part of Policy Review

Some committees rarely write policy (either because they do not choose to or because they are in an institution in which policy writing belongs somewhere else in the organizational chart), but are expected to review policies when they are written. In theory, this is a good choice for those who find policy writing a time-consuming and unproductive use of committee time. Reviewing policy, however, has its own set of problems. For the committee to report back that policy A "does not deal adequately with informed consent" may not be very helpful to the original policy writer; on the other hand, drafting specific language puts the committee in the business of writing policy in a forum that may not be very conducive to the activity. In addition, the committee may suggest changes but never know what happened next, because the policy is unlikely to be sent back and forth for review repeatedly. (It is easy to imagine a situation in which the committee repeatedly does not like the way the policy writer handles informed consent and the policy writer does not know what to do to satisfy the committee. At such times, the aphorism "if you want something done right, do it yourself" comes quickly to mind.) If the ethics committee is to review policy but not make revisions, there should be some mechanism by which it is at least informed about the final policy decisions.

Fitting the Approach to the Committee's Culture

In deciding how to approach policy writing, the committee leadership needs to think about the characteristics of its committee and what approach suits it best. It is possible to mix these models—sometimes working with the whole committee, sometimes using a subcommittee, or sometimes just reviewing others' work. Making this decision thoughtfully and providing whoever is writing the draft with clear guidelines on policy scope and time constraints is important.

The Policy-Writing Process

Giving structure to the policy-writing process will help keep it from consuming all the committee's energy. The most difficult part of being the chairperson of a committee (or of a subcommittee) working on policy may be knowing when to say "Enough!" and when to say "Let's extend this discussion to the next meeting."

Those directing policy writing should consider devoting a meeting or two to identifying the central substantive issues the policy should resolve. After that, the policy's language can be drafted (this is either done from scratch or by drawing on policies written by another facility). Assigning the actual writing of the draft to one person and having that person be responsible for incorporating the changes of multiple drafts helps to create some kind of responsible continuity. This will work only if the committee has a member who is a good synthesizer; that is, someone who is able to take on the responsibility for incorporating others' views into a single document rather than impressing his or her own views on the document. If the primary drafter sees the document as his or her own work, there is always the risk of defensiveness when anyone suggests changing it. Ownership of the policy must ultimately go to the committee. A committee that has a good sense of itself as a community will have an easier time of it than will a committee of individualists.

It is helpful to have the final version of policies in the following form: (1) a summary statement of the policy, (2) a list of critical terms and their definitions, (3) a list of the principles that form the ethical foundation of the policy, and (4) the procedures to be followed for the discrete sections of the policy. In the policy review previously referred to, the most significant problem was an absence of definitions.

Those drafting a policy should start by writing a single statement summarizing the policy. Continued work should not proceed until the drafting group agrees that this statement incorporates all that the policy hopes to achieve. Then the drafter should extract all the terms from that statement that are open to interpretation and use them as the basis of a definition list.

A well-drafted policy summary statement should contain all the critical concepts of the policy. The principles should include all statements relating to the facility's beliefs and values that shape this policy. The statement of principles need not be articulated in the language of philosophy; that is, a statement that "patients have the right to make their own treatment decisions" implies the principle of autonomy without stating it. Using plain language is always better. Procedures sections of policies need to be broken up into subgroups, for example, health care provider responsibilities, determinations of decision-making capacity, identification of surrogates, resolution of disagreements, documentation requirements, and so forth. Often, the procedures section of a policy jumbles many things together with no clear organization. Think of actually going through the procedure: what do you need to do first? Second? What do you do if you have done all this and there is still conflict? (The last section of the procedures section should address conflict resolution.) Some committees include references to authoritative documents and law in their policies, others do not. (See figure 6-1 for an example of a policy statement for life-sustaining treatment decisions.)

Education on Policies

Although committees spend a lot of time writing policies, they are often reluctant to provide education on those policies. This is discouraging to those who have worked hard to get the policy written and makes members feel that policy making (and perhaps the committee itself) is no more than busywork. Ethics committee members are often reluctant to put themselves forward as teachers in any kind of formal setting. Perhaps this results from the fear that others will perceive them as trying to assert moral superiority. Only in a few committees that we have observed has there been successful interdisciplinary education on policy. That is, seldom are nurses successfully involved in helping physicians understand a new or revised policy, although physicians are perhaps more frequently involved in teaching nurses. Members are more comfortable "teaching their own" than teaching others.

This difficulty in conducting education on policy may arise from the fact that the ethics committee (as previously noted) understands the policy as a process, which is different from the way others in the institution view the policy; for example, the ethics committee may want to discuss how to *think* about the issue whereas the clinician will want to know what he or she can or cannot *do*. This is a big gap to overcome. To do this kind of education successfully, the committee must accept the clinician's perspective as legitimate. The gap between these two perspectives may be bridged by beginning with cases in which the policy is easily applied and then working up to those in which application is more complex.

The committee might also try to view education as more than giving lectures. For example, policies or summaries could be published in newsletters or pamphlets and then distributed throughout the facility; the committee could sponsor brown-bag lunches where people could meet to talk about the policy in the context of a particular case; or the committee could conduct meetings with various groups in the process of writing the policy to obtain their views on specific points. This last strategy can be very helpful in a number of ways. First, it tells people in advance that changes are being considered and it asks them to contribute to the changes. (Anesthesiologists and surgeons, for example, have been very helpful—indeed essential—to most committees that have involved them in the revision of DNR policies to incorporate DNR in surgery.) Second, those closest to the cases that will be affected by the policy often have perspectives on practical problems that the committee may not fully understand. (For example, ICU nurses have alerted ethics committees to their uncertainty about the meaning of DNR orders when a monitored patient experiences bradycardia. Does the DNR order mean that lidocaine should or should not be used?) If, however, the committee does not plan to engage in any education on policy outside the committee, it should skip policy writing entirely (unless someone else in the institution is planning to take on the educational aspects of the task).

Figure 6-1. Life-Sustaining Treatment Decisions: Sample Statement of Policy

Adult patients with decision-making capacity, after being given adequate information on treatment and after having received a recommendation on treatment from their primary physician or consultant, shall be the final decision maker as to whether they wish to accept or refuse any or all treatment that their primary or consulting physician believes is medically appropriate for their condition. A surrogate shall be identified for adult patients who lack decision-making capacity, and the surrogate shall consent to or refuse treatment for the patient in accordance with any advance directive given by the patient and under the same conditions that the adult patient with decision-making capacity would give consent or refusal. Minors (children and adolescents) should be encouraged to participate in their treatment decisions to the extent that they have the capacity to do so. Medically appropriate life-sustaining treatment shall be provided to any patient (including a minor) who requests it.

How to Evaluate a Policy

Evaluation of new policies can be conducted in many ways. Some committees have been able to conduct policy evaluation by involving quality assurance groups in the monitoring of discrete aspects of the policy. Others have done chart review (which is a time-consuming activity). Committees might try to ascertain whether staff and physicians know about the existence of the policy or its acceptability by surveys. For example, the committee might have a physician member arrange to distribute and collect a very short questionnaire during a medical staff meeting; enlist the support of nursing directors and social service directors in surveying nurses or nurse supervisors and social workers; or publish a short questionnaire in the institutional newsletter.

Conclusion

Many people on ethics committees believe that policies are largely unknown in hospitals and, if known, are largely ignored—that is, that they exist to satisfy regulators and to make hospital attorneys sleep better. This may reflect reality, but it need not permanently define reality. In the years to come, hospitals will increasingly be expected to understand and articulate their standards and it is to their policies that they must look to find this articulation.

Ethics committees would be missing an important aspect of their role if they ignored policy writing entirely. However, policy writing, even more than case review and education, requires a full commitment to be meaningful. Thus, members and committee leaders should think carefully about whether policy writing is what they *want* to do. Those who determine the committee's scope of authority should think carefully about whether policy writing is what they want from their committee. It may be appropriate for those who determine the committee's authority and the committee leadership to discuss together whether and how the committee should view hospital policy formulation. If it is to be done well, ultimately it will require more resources than the committee can provide on its own.

Exercises

1. Look at your DNR, forgoing treatment, or other relevant policy.
   - Is CPR defined? For example, when there is a written DNR order, the health care professional is not to perform CPR. What is it that he or she is or is not supposed to do? Does everyone agree? It is surprising how little agreement exists on the boundaries of CPR.
   - What does your policy advise you to do if the patient lacks decision-making capacity and has no surrogate?
   - What does your policy advise if the physician thinks that the patient lacks decision-making capacity but the patient or family member disagrees?
   - What does your policy advise if there is disagreement among family members on who speaks for the patient?
   - What does your policy say about informing nursing staff about patients' DNR decisions? Is it enough that physicians inform nurses that the patient/surrogate wants a DNR order, or do physicians also have to explain the rationale for the order?
   - What does your policy say about physicians' objections of conscience? About nurses' objections of conscience?
   - If a patient with a DNR order has a cardiac arrest in the course of a procedure (either in the operating room, in the ICU, or on the floor), does your policy explain what should be done?
   - What does your policy advise if families insist that the patient not be given information, especially if the family is from a culture that does not espouse individual autonomy in the way that the dominant U.S. culture does?
2. Obtain policies from another institution that are on the same topic as those written by your ethics committee. Compare discrete sections of the two (about a half-page worth, for example). Are they different? Is the difference substantive? Which do you prefer?

3. Have committee members list all known existing hospital policies that they believe are related to bioethics. Is there agreement on what policies are most affected by bioethics?

4. Ask each member to state what hospital policy is most important from his or her perspective and to explain that perspective (for example, very common issue, issue that is frequently handled poorly, supports them in getting colleagues to deal appropriately with patients, and so on). Ask members if there is a policy that does not exist but that they wish did.

5. Draw a flowchart for an existing policy. Does information in this format make it easier to understand the policy? (See the treatment decisions flowchart in appendix 6-2.)

Notes and References

1. One article that committees would be advised to read on this topic provides a detailed description of a committee's efforts/struggles to create a policy dealing with treating patients who are Jehovah's Witnesses and who refuse life-sustaining blood transfusions. See: Macklin, R. The inner workings of an ethics committee: latest battle of Jehovah's Witnesses. *Hastings Center Report* 18(1):15–20, 1988.

2. Reports of The President's Commission for the Study of Ethical Issues in Medicine and Biomedical and Behavioral Research, particularly: *Deciding to Forego Life-Sustaining Treatment* (1983), *Defining Death* (1981), and *Making Health Care Decisions,* 3 vols. (1982–1983), Washington, DC: U.S. Government Printing Office.

3. *Guidelines on the Termination of Life-Sustaining Treatment and the Care of the Dying.* A report by The Hastings Center. Briarcliff Manor, NY: The Hastings Center, 1987.

4. *Appleton Suggested International Guidelines for Decisions to Forego Medical Treatment.* Lawrence University Program in Bioethics. Appleton, WI: Lawrence University, 1988.

5. *American College of Physicians Ethics Manual.* 3rd ed. As published in: *Annals of Internal Medicine* 117(11):947–60, 1992.

6. Joint Los Angeles County Bar Association and Los Angeles County Medical Association Committee on Biomedical Ethics. Guidelines for foregoing life-sustaining treatment for adult patients. *Los Angeles Lawyer,* July 1990, pp. 24–27, 41–43.

7. Wenger, N., Young, R., and Ross, J. W. An ethics committee's recommendations on testing patients for HIV antibodies when health care workers suffer exposure to blood-borne pathogens. *HEC Forum* 3(6):329–36, 1991.

8. Miles, S. New business for ethics committees. *HEC Forum* 4(2):97–102, 1992.

Appendix 6-1. Sample Policies: CPR and Futility

CPR Policy

Policy
The option of cardiopulmonary resuscitation (CPR) will be offered to all patients who are at risk for cardiac or pulmonary arrest and for whom it may be effective. If the patient/surrogate consents to CPR, the physician will write a CPR order. If CPR will not be effective or if the patient/surrogate refuses CPR, the physician will write a "no CPR" order.

Principles
1. Patients with decision-making capacity have the right to consent to or to refuse any medical treatment that is offered to them.
2. Physicians have a duty to judge whether medical treatment offers the patient more than a minimal possibility of benefit and, if it does, to offer it to the patient, or to the surrogate if the patient lacks decision-making capacity. The physician also has a duty to recommend a course of action to the patient or the surrogate decision maker.
3. Patients or their surrogate decision makers are entitled to know when a relevant treatment is judged not to have minimal benefit and to obtain a second opinion from a physician of their choice about that judgment.
4. All members of the health care team should be knowledgeable about any decisions to withhold or provide treatment.
5. Family members, significant others, or close friends are appropriate surrogate decision makers for patients who lack decision-making capacity unless they are clearly not acting in compliance with the patient's previously expressed wishes or, if they are not known, the patient's best interests.
6. Adolescents who are capable of participating in treatment decisions should be involved in those decisions, along with their parents/guardians.
7. Patients are entitled to be told the truth about their condition, their prognosis, and the probable outcome of treatment that is available to them, unless they ask not to be given that information. In such a case, the information should be provided to a surrogate decision maker.
8. A patient's clearly expressed advance directive is to be respected by the health care team.
9. Patients are to be treated fairly with respect to judgments about possible treatment benefit and effectiveness. A judgment that treatment will provide benefit or be effective will be made as objectively as possible and without consideration of the patient's quality of life or personal, nonmedically relevant characteristics, except that benefits shall require that there be a potential for the patient of positive response to his/her environment.

Definitions
1. *CPR:* In the acute care setting, CPR includes all elements of advanced CPR that are available and potentially effective in restoring cardiac or pulmonary function after cardiac or pulmonary arrest has occurred.
2. *Consent:* The patient's or surrogate's consent or refusal must be informed. That is, he/she must be provided with adequate information about potential need for treatment, risks and benefits of treatment, alternatives to treatment, and risks of receiving no treatment.
3. *CPR and "No CPR" order:* A written order to initiate or not to initiate CPR in the event of cardiac or pulmonary arrest.
4. *Benefit (to patient):* Refers to outcomes that can be experienced by the patient in a positive way. In the case of CPR, conscious life extended beyond minutes/hours is considered to be a benefit.
5. *Decision-making capacity:* A patient's ability to understand the need for treatment, the risks and benefit of having or refusing treatment, and alternatives to treatment, and to make a considered decision about treatment based on this information and on personal values.
6. *Surrogate decision maker:* Any individual who may or may not be legally related to a patient who lacks decision-making capacity, but who has had an ongoing relationship with the patient so that she/he is able to understand the patient's values and probable choices is a potential surrogate decision maker.
7. *Best interests:* A judgment made by a physician or surrogate that a treatment is proportionate; that is, that its benefits to the patient outweigh its burdens to the patient.
8. *Advance directive:* Any written or oral statement by the patient that specifies what treatment the patient would want in the future.
9. *Minimal possibility of benefit:* A judgment that the statistical probability of benefit of CPR is very small; approaching zero.

Procedures

I. The physician shall determine whether CPR has the possibility of minimal benefit for any patient who is at risk of suffering cardiac or pulmonary arrest.

    A. If the decision is that there is no minimum probability of benefit:

        1. The physician shall explain that judgment to the patient or surrogate decision maker and permit them to obtain a second opinion from a physician of the patient's choice as to possible benefit.

        2. If the patient/surrogate does not choose to obtain a second opinion, the physician shall explain this decision to other members of the health care team, write a "no CPR" order in the patient's chart, and complete the appropriate documentation.

        3. If the patient/surrogate wishes a second opinion and that second physician concludes that CPR has a minimum probability of benefit, then the patient will be offered CPR.

        4. If the second physician concludes that CPR does not offer a minimal possibility of benefit, then the patient/surrogate may be offered the option of transferring the patient to another facility.

    B. If the decision is that there is more than a minimum probability of benefit:

        1. The physician shall explain to the patient/surrogate the potential benefit and probable risks of CPR for this patient and shall offer a recommendation.

        2. The patient/surrogate shall determine the relative importance of risks and benefits and consequently whether she/he will accept or refuse CPR.

        3. If the patient refuses CPR, the physician, with the patient's consent, will discuss with family members the patient's decision to refuse CPR and will explain to the family the implications of that decision.

II. Regarding surrogate decision makers:

    A. The physician shall determine whether a patient has decision-making capacity and whether a surrogate decision maker is required by the patient, consulting as needed other members of the health care team. If there is uncertainty or disagreement about the patient's decision-making capacity, consultation from other specialties (psychiatry, neurology, for example) should be sought.

    B. If a surrogate decision maker is required, it shall be the person designated by the patient in a durable power of attorney for health care, a legally appointed conservator, or a person named in any other advance directive.

    C. If there is more than one potential surrogate decision maker, no one of whom the patient has previously designated as the chosen surrogate, the physician shall request that the potential surrogates determine who among them should be the designated surrogate for the patient.

    D. If there is disagreement among potential surrogate decision makers about who should be the patient's surrogate or about what course of treatment should be followed, ethics committee review should be offered. Court resolution via conservatorship proceedings should be sought only if conflict is irresolvable.

III. If members of the health care team disagree about the validity or appropriateness of a patient's decision to refuse CPR, resolution shall be sought at the unit level or through an ethics committee review.

IV. Regarding objections of conscience:

    A. A physician who objects as a matter of conscience to writing a "no CPR" order requested by a patient or to the patient's refusal of a recommended DNR order shall transfer the care of the patient to a physician who will accept the patient's wishes.

    B. A physician who objects as a matter of conscience to a surrogate's decision to consent to or to refuse a DNR order when there is no clear evidence of the patient's wishes shall request ethics committee review or shall transfer the care of the patient to a physician who will abide by the surrogate's decision.

V. Documentation: Physicians shall document the decision to write or not to write a "no CPR" order as follows:

    A. Basis of the decision that CPR will or will not offer minimum benefit to the patient.

    B. Discussion with patient/surrogate of that judgment, including the patient's/surrogate's desire for a second opinion, or the patient's decision to consent to or refuse CPR.

    C. Description of the patient's capacity for decision making.

    D. Physician's recommendations regarding CPR.

    E. Identification of surrogate, if indicated.

    F. Basis for surrogate's decision regarding a "no CPR" order.

    G. Existence of advance directives. (Copy to be included in chart, if written directive.)

VI. Both CPR and "no CPR" orders must be written by the physician. If accepted over the telephone, the call must be witnessed and written documentation provided within 24 hours.

VII. Review of CPR and "no CPR" orders.
  A. All orders to provide or forgo CPR shall be reviewed whenever there is a change in the patient's condition.
  B. All members of the health care team have a duty to draw the physician's attention to any change in the patient's condition that requires review of the patient's CPR status.

VIII. Special Situations:
  A. Surgery: A patient who has a "no CPR" order may still be an appropriate candidate for palliative surgery. Prior to the proposed surgery, the attending physician shall inform the surgeon of the patient's "no CPR" order, and the surgeon or anesthesiologist shall discuss with the patient/surrogate the risks and benefits of the "no CPR" order during surgery. Patient/surrogate and physicians shall come to agreement about how the "no CPR" order is to be handled in the course of surgery and immediate postsurgical recovery. In the surgical context, a distinction is to be made between cardiac arrest and pulmonary arrest insofar as pulmonary arrest will be treated since it is a concomitant of the anesthesia. The surgeon or anesthesiologist shall document the discussion and the decision about resuscitation status for the surgery patient.
  B. Adolescents: Although adolescents (other than emancipated minors) may not legally consent to or refuse treatment, they should be a party to all decisions about CPR and their assent sought.
  C. Children or infants: Parents/guardians are the appropriate decision makers for infants and children. If they appear not to be acting in their child's or infant's best interests, ethics committee review should be sought.
  D. Religious exceptions: Patients whose refusal of treatment is based on unusual religious views should be engaged in conversation to ensure that they understand the implications of their views. If they understand, their views should be respected.
  E. Transfer of patients: Patients who have a "no CPR" order and who are to be transferred to other facilities should be accompanied by specific documentation of the "no CPR" order.
  F. Emergency room reception of patients with "no CPR" or "DNR" orders: If the patient is admitted to the emergency room with a "no CPR" or a DNR order and identification recognized by this hospital, CPR shall not be performed unless requested by the patient.
  G. If a patient has requested a "no CPR" order and, at the time of arrest, family members urge that resuscitation be performed, CPR will not be performed.

Source: Center for Healthcare Ethics, a service of St. Joseph Health System, Orange, CA.

DNR Policy

Cardiopulmonary resuscitation (CPR) will be given to any patient who suffers cardiac or pulmonary arrest unless the attending physician has previously written a do-not-resuscitate (DNR) order or is present at the time of the arrest and gives oral orders not to perform CPR.

Principles
1. Patients with decision-making capacity have the right to consent to or refuse any medical treatment that is offered to them.
2. Physicians have a duty to discuss with seriously ill patients who are at risk of cardiopulmonary arrest the patient's preferences about receiving CPR. The physician also has a duty to recommend accepting or forgoing resuscitation to the patient or, if the patient lacks decision-making capacity, to the surrogate decision maker.
3. All members of the health care team have a duty to communicate information relevant to resuscitation and patients' wishes to the physician, and a duty to be knowledgeable about decisions to withhold CPR.
4. Family members, significant others, or close friends are appropriate surrogate decision makers for patients who lack decision-making capacity unless they are clearly not acting in compliance with the patient's previously expressed wishes or, if these wishes are not known, the patient's best interests.
5. Adolescents and children who are capable of participating in treatment decisions should be involved in those decisions, along with their parents/guardians.
6. Patients are entitled to be told the truth about their condition, their prognosis, and the probable outcome of treatment recommendations, unless they ask not to be given that information. In such a case, the information would be provided to a surrogate decision maker.
7. A patient's clearly expressed advance directive is to be respected by the health care team.
8. Health care professionals should not be expected to act in violation of their personal moral values.
9. Treatment that cannot be expected to provide any benefit to the patient need not be offered.

Definitions
1. *CPR:* In the acute care setting, CPR includes all elements of basic and advanced CPR that are available and potentially effective in restoring cardiac or pulmonary function after cardiac or pulmonary arrest has occurred.
2. *DNR:* A physician's written order not to initiate CPR in the event of cardiac or pulmonary arrest.
3. *Benefit (to the patient):* Outcomes that can be experienced by the patient in a positive way. In the case of CPR, conscious life extended beyond minutes/hours is considered to be a benefit. However, only the patient/surrogate can decide whether the benefit is sufficient to offset the risks and burdens of resuscitation and continued life.
4. *Decision-making capacity:* A patient's ability to understand the need for treatment, as well as the risks and benefits of having or refusing treatment, and to make a considered decision about treatment based on this information and on personal values.
5. *Surrogate decision maker:* Any designated individual who may or may not be legally related to a patient who lacks decision-making capacity, but who has had an ongoing relationship with the patient so that he/she has some understanding of the patient's values and probable choices.
6. *Best interests:* A judgment made by a physician or surrogate that a treatment is proportionate; that is, that its benefits to the patient outweigh its burdens to the patient.
7. *Advance directive:* Any written or oral statement by the patient that specifies what treatment the patient would want in the future or that names a person to be the recognized decision maker should the patient become decisionally incapacitated.

Procedures
1. The physician shall determine whether a patient is at risk of cardiopulmonary arrest, and whether there is any probability that the patient will benefit from resuscitation.
2. If there is a risk and no probability of benefit to the patient, the physician shall write a DNR order and inform the patient/surrogate of this order.
3. If there is such a risk and there is a probable benefit, the physician shall determine whether the patient has the capacity to decide about receiving CPR.
4. If the patient does have decision-making capacity:
   A. The physician shall discuss the use of CPR with the patient, and make a recommendation about the use of CPR.

B. If the patient wishes resuscitation, no DNR order will be written. If the patient does not wish resuscitation in the event of cardiopulmonary arrest, the physician shall write a DNR order in the patient's chart and complete appropriate documentation.

C. With the patient's consent, the physician will discuss with family members the patient's decision not to receive CPR and will explain to the family the implications of that decision.

5. If the patient does not have decision-making capacity:
   A. The physician shall determine who is an appropriate surrogate decision-maker. (See 6, following.)
   B. The physician shall discuss the use of CPR with the surrogate, determine whether the patient's previous wishes are known, and make a recommendation about the use of CPR.
   C. If the physician advises no resuscitation and the surrogate decision maker consents to a DNR order, the physician shall write a DNR order in the patient's chart and complete the appropriate documentation.
   D. If the surrogate decision maker and the physician disagree about whether the patient should receive CPR and the patient's wishes are not known, ethics committee review shall be sought.

6. Designation of surrogate decision maker.
   A. If a surrogate decision maker is required, it shall be the person designated by the patient in a durable power of attorney for health care or a comparable advance directive, or a conservator if there is a conservator and the conservator has medical decision-making authority.
   B. If there is more than one potential surrogate decision maker, no one of whom has previously been designated by the patient as the chosen surrogate, the physician shall request that they determine who among them shall be the patient's surrogate decision maker.
   C. If there is disagreement among potential surrogate decision makers about who should be the patient's surrogate, or if the physician believes that the family's decision about who should be the surrogate is inappropriate, ethics committee assistance should be sought.
   D. If agreement cannot be reached about a surrogate decision maker and there is disagreement among potential surrogates about the appropriate course of treatment, court appointment of a conservator may need to be sought.

7. If members of the health care team disagree about the validity or appropriateness of a patient's decision to refuse CPR, resolution shall be sought at the unit level or through an ethics committee review.

8. Objections of conscience.
   A. A physician who objects as a matter of conscience to writing a DNR order requested by a patient or to the patient's refusal of a recommended DNR order shall transfer the care of the patient to a physician who will abide by the patient's wishes, if such a physician is available.
   B. A physician who objects as a matter of conscience to a surrogate's decision to consent to or refuse a DNR order when there is no clear evidence of the patient's wishes shall request ethics committee review or shall transfer the care of the patient to a physician who will abide by the surrogate's decision, if such a physician is available.
   C. All members of the health care team should understand the reasons for providing or withholding CPR.

9. Documentation: Physicians shall document the decision to write a DNR order as follows:
   A. Diagnosis, prognosis, probable response to CPR. If CPR is thought to provide no benefit for the patient, the reasons for that judgment shall be documented, as well as the discussion with the patient/surrogate about that decision.
   B. Assessment of patient's decision-making capacity.
   C. Reasons for patient's decision to consent to a DNR order.
   D. Identification of surrogate (if indicated).
   E. Reasons for surrogate's decision about a DNR order.
   F. Existence of advance directives. (Written advance directives should be placed in chart. Oral directives shall be documented.)
   G. Orders for forgoing prearrest treatment, if appropriate (for example, treatment for hypotension, bradycardia, ventricular tachycardia, or respiratory insufficiency). (See 13.H, following.)
   H. Supportive care orders, if appropriate.

10. DNR orders must be written. If accepted over the telephone, the call must be witnessed and countersigned within 48 hours.

11. Review of DNR orders.
    A. All DNR orders shall be reviewed whenever there is a change in the patient's condition, change in the attending physician, or change in the unit of the health care facility.
    B. All members of the health care team have a duty to inform the physician if they believe there is a reason for review of a DNR order.

C. If a patient orally rescinds or questions a DNR order, this should be immediately brought to the attention of the attending physician, and documented in the order sheet and progress notes.

12. If the patient is transferred to another unit or to another facility, appropriate documentation of the DNR order shall accompany the patient.

13. Special Situations:

A. Surgery: A patient who has a DNR order may still be an appropriate candidate for surgery (for example, palliative surgery). Prior to the proposed surgery, the attending physician shall inform the surgeon of the patient's DNR order, and the surgeon or anesthesiologist shall discuss with the patient/surrogate the risks and benefits of the DNR order during surgery. They and the patient/surrogate shall reach consensus as to how the DNR order is to be handled in the course of surgery and during immediate postsurgical recovery. In the context of general anesthesia, a distinction is to be made between cardiac arrest and pulmonary arrest insofar as pulmonary arrest will be treated since it is a concomitant of general anesthesia. The surgeon or anesthesiologist shall document the decision about resuscitation status for the surgery patient and the reasons for either continuing the DNR order or revoking it during the surgery and immediate postsurgery period. No member of the health care team who objects as a matter of conscience to a decision to maintain a DNR order during surgery shall be required to participate in the surgical procedure.

B. Adolescents: Although adolescents (other than emancipated minors) may not legally consent to or refuse treatment, they should be a party to all decisions about CPR and their assent sought.

C. Children or infants: Parents/guardians are almost always the appropriate decision makers for infants and children. If they appear not to be acting in their child's or infant's best interest, ethics committee review should be sought.

D. Religious and philosophical exceptions: Patients whose refusal of treatment is based on religious or personal philosophic views should be engaged in conversation to ensure that they understand the implications of their views. If they do understand, their views should be respected, unless their decision endangers others who are dependent on them. In such situations, ethics committee review shall be sought.

E. Emergency room reception of patients with DNR orders: If the patient is admitted to the emergency room with a DNR order and identification is recognized by this hospital, CPR shall not be performed unless there is convincing evidence that DNR is inappropriate.

G. If a patient has requested a DNR order and, at the time of arrest, family members urge that resuscitation be performed, CPR will not be performed unless there is reason to believe the patient would wish it to be.

H. Prearrest treatment: If a patient with a DNR order experiences prearrest symptoms, he/she shall be provided with standard forms of treatment unless the physician has specifically ordered that such treatment shall not be provided (for example, ventilation for respiratory distress, treatment of hypotension, bradycardia, or ventricular tachycardia).

I. Patients who lack decision-making capacity and have no surrogates: Patients who need but have no surrogate have the same right as other patients with respect to refusing CPR. If the physician determines that a DNR order would serve the best interests of such a patient, the decision should be reviewed by the entire health care team or by an ethics committee, and the reasons for the order and the review process should be carefully documented. In some cases, it may be appropriate for the hospital to initiate conservatorship proceedings.

14. A decision not to provide CPR does not mean that any other form of treatment is to be withheld. For example, palliative treatments (including surgery) to reduce or eliminate pain and suffering or to improve levels of functioning may be indicated. The patient should never be made to feel that a decision not to receive CPR results in being abandoned by health care professionals.

15. Partial codes: If CPR is to be effective, all aspects of it should be used. However, very occasionally it may be appropriate to restrict some aspects of CPR, when honoring a patient's request for a partial or limited code. When a partial or limited order for CPR is written, the physician shall document the reasons for this limitation.

16. Slow codes: Slow codes are deceptive and are intended to be deceptive and thus are never appropriate.

17. Conflict resolution regarding DNR orders: Disputes concerning DNR orders should be discussed with the attending physician and, if unresolved, with other hospital authorities or the ethics committee.

Source: Center for Healthcare Ethics, a service of St. Joseph Health System, Orange, CA.

Executive Committee Policy for Withholding or Withdrawing Futile Treatments

Philosophy of Care

The primary goals of the physician are to promote healing, to prevent disease, to forestall untimely death, and to relieve suffering. When possible, the physician should treat to cure and bring about full functional recovery. However, when the patient's disease process or injury overmatches medicine's ability to bring about recovery, the physician should offer palliation for the patient's discomfort and help the patient cope with illness, disability, and dying.

In pursuing these medical goals, the physician must observe several professional duties. They include the duty to respect the patient's dignity and autonomy, to uphold the ethical principles of medicine, and to observe professional standards of practice. Taken together, these duties suggest a partnership between physician and patient regulated by the ethical principles of shared decision making and mutual respect.

The principle of shared decision making secures to the patient rights of informed consent or informed refusal of treatment. Correlative with these rights are the physician's obligations to inform the patient about his or her medical condition, prognosis, and treatment options together with their likely risks and benefits. The care offered to the patient should reflect the physician's best medical judgment and conform to professional standards. Although the decision whether to refuse or to accept any treatment, including life-sustaining treatment, ultimately belongs to the patient, the principle of mutual respect implies that neither the physician nor the patient may reduce the other to a mere instrument of will. The physician must respect the patient's right to refuse offers of treatment as well as to accept them. The patient should respect that it is the physician's responsibility to determine the appropriate treatment options from which he or she may choose.

In the face of terminal illness or potentially fatal injury, observing these ethical requirements is especially important. The patient's disease, injury, or treatment itself may deprive the patient of capacity to exercise directly his or her rights to informed consent or informed refusal. If a terminally, incurably ill patient loses decision-making capacity and has made it clear by written or by oral declarations that he or she wants not to be kept alive by extraordinary means or by artificial nutrition and hydration, then consistent with good medical practice, the patient's wishes should be honored. If the patient has a living will or has executed a health care power of attorney, then these expressions of the patient's wishes should be respected as authoritative.

In the absence of formal evidence of the patient's wishes, it is customary and appropriate to rely on the patient's spouse, close family member(s), or other person(s) with fair claim to best represent the patient in decision making. Whoever bears the responsibility for exercising the patient's rights of informed consent or informed refusal of treatment should regulate his or her decision-making role by the doctrines of *substituted judgment* or of *best interest*.

Under the doctrine of substituted judgment, the patient's representative attempts to determine whether the patient would have consented to or refused treatment by reference to the patient's expressed wishes, value system, or other reliable evidence of the patient's wishes. If no such evidence exists, the patient's representative should consider accepting or rejecting treatments by appeal to the patient's best interest, that is, by asking what a reasonable person would want for himself or herself were he or she in the patient's circumstances.

Such contingencies notwithstanding, it remains the physician's responsibility to offer an optimum care plan that responds to changes in the patient's condition and accords with professional standards of practice.

When any intervention, including those that are life-sustaining, (a) fails to hold a reasonable promise for bringing about the patient's recovery, (b) imposes burdens grossly disproportional to any expectable patient benefit, (c) plays no effective role in mitigating the patient's discomfort, and (d) serves only to postpone artificially the moment of death by sustaining, supplanting, or restoring a vital function, then the intervention is medically futile and there is no obligation to offer to initiate it, or to offer to continue it.

Should the patient's attending physician determine that any intervention meets these criteria, he or she should communicate this promptly to the patient or to the patient's representative(s). The patient and/or the patient's representative(s) should understand and concur with the decision to withhold or withdraw medically futile interventions. However, neither the patient nor the patient's representative may compel the physician to act contrary to his or her best medical judgment.*

The following describes an *optional, nonexclusive* procedure whereby life-sustaining interventions may be withheld or withdrawn from a terminally, incurably ill patient† on grounds that such measures hold no reasonable promise to benefit the patient medically. Nothing in this policy infringes or impairs any right of the patient or any responsibility of the patient's physician.

1. When the patient's attending physician determines that the patient's medical condition is terminal, and incurable, and;

2. When the patient's attending physician determines that available interventions hold no reasonable promise to benefit the patient medically; that is, available interventions (1) hold no reasonable promise for contributing to or for bringing about the patient's recovery, (2) would impose burdens grossly disproportionate to any expected patient benefit, (3) would fail to palliate the patient's discomfort, and (4) would serve only to postpone artificially the moment of death by sustaining, supplanting, or restoring a vital function and;

3. When the patient's attending physician documents these judgments in the patient's medical record, then;

4. The patient's attending physician is under no obligation to initiate or to continue such interventions.

5. When a patient's attending physician determines that the patient's medical condition is terminal, and incurable, and proposes to withhold or to withdraw any intervention including life-saving or life-sustaining measures on the grounds mentioned in number 2, and has documented these determinations in the patient's medical record, then the attending physician promptly shall so inform the patient or his or her representative(s). The patient or his or her representative(s) shall enjoy the opportunity to secure the services of another physician, or otherwise to arrange transfer of the patient to another health care provider, if desired.

6. If the patient's attending physician obtains the concurrence of the cognizant ethics committee, then the determinations made by such physician in accordance with the policy shall be deemed to have been made pursuant to, and in full compliance with, the policies and procedures of the Charlotte-Mecklenburg Hospital Authority.

Notes

*Current American Medical Association guidelines for the appropriate use of DNR orders address physicians' obligations to offer futile interventions in a manner entirely consistent with the policy recommendations herein. "A physician is not ethically obligated to make a specific diagnostic or therapeutic procedure available to a patient even on specific request, if the use of such a procedure would be futile." [Council on Ethical and Judicial Affairs. Guidelines for the appropriate use of do-not-resuscitate orders. *JAMA* 1991;265;1868–1971].

†"Terminally and incurably ill" means the patient suffers from an illness (1) for which no known measures are effective in reversing its course, (2) whose course has progressed beyond the capacity of existing knowledge and technique to stem or arrest it, and (3) which would result in death within days or weeks unless *extraordinary means* are used. "Extraordinary means" refers to any medical procedure or intervention that in the judgment of the attending physician would serve only to postpone artificially the moment of death by sustaining, restoring, or supplanting a vital function.

Reprinted, with permission, from the Carolinas Medical Center, Charlotte, NC. Copyright 1992.

The Parkland Approach to Demands for "Futile" Treatment

Key words: Futility, DNR (or Do Not Resuscitate), CPR (or Cardiopulmonary Resuscitation), Autonomy, Life-Sustaining Treatment.

Approach

If a competent patient or the family or surrogate of an incompetent patient requests or demands a "life-saving" or "life-preserving" treatment, and the attending physician is of the opinion that the treatment is useless and without benefit, the physician should take the following steps:

A. Consult the Institutional Ethics Committee.

B. Consult two (2) physicians from a relevant specialty to render an opinion about the usefulness of the disputed treatment. The consultants should enter their opinion in the progress notes within 24 hours of receipt of the attending physicians' notice.

C. If the Institutional Ethics Committee has been consulted and the attending physician and both consultants are unanimous in their opinion of the uselessness or futility of the disputed treatment, the treatment should not be provided.

D. If for some reason the conditions in A, B, and C above have not or cannot be met, the disputed treatment should be administered until these conditions have been met.

E. Providing or denying a disputed treatment should not affect the provision of other treatments that benefit the patient.

Discussion

The Institutional Ethics Committee's including a section on futility reflected a number of concerns. Some members of the medical staff wanted the hospital administration to acknowledge explicitly the role of physician authority and autonomy in providing beneficial treatment. This concern was met simply by including a discussion of the futility issue in the guidelines. Second, Parkland Memorial Hospital is a public hospital that serves a large indigent population. Thus, it is often the hospital of only resort for many of its patients. For those patients, disputes over treatment can mean the difference between some treatment and no treatment at all. Third, the Committee sought to protect the interests of patients in disputes over this category of treatment preference. These latter two concerns raise more subtle and vexing issues.

The Committee decided that it would be a mistake to draft its guidelines around any one definition of futility. We concluded from our review of the futility literature that any particular definition tacitly protected certain value judgments and rejected others. By contrast, a consensus-based approach to dealing with futility respects differences among patients and practitioners and deals more effectively with context and nuance. In addition, any single definition of futility would have precluded the level of support necessary for administrative and medical staff approval.

The Committee also recognized that disputes over the efficacy of treatment can occur between physicians and that scientific medicine seldom is definitive. Patient demands for particular treatments seem most entitled to respect when there is a disagreement among physicians over efficacy. For this reason, the Committee established unanimity among three physicians as the standard for determinations of futility. This standard broadly protects patient authority to request treatments of questionable efficacy. It also preserves the physician's choice to not provide treatments that are clearly without benefit. The high standard, along with the requirement for ethics committee consultation, is particularly appropriate for a patient population with limited, often nonexistent, alternatives for care.

Reprinted, with permission, from John Z. Sadler, M.D., and Thomas W. Mayo, J.D., The Institutional Ethics Committee, Parkland Memorial Hospital, Dallas County Hospital District.

Appendix 6-2. Flowchart of Making Treatment Decisions

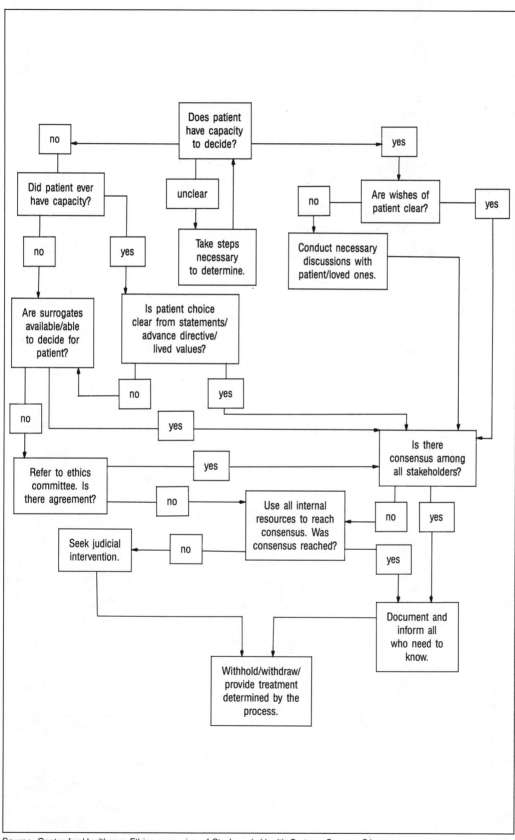

Source: Center for Healthcare Ethics, a service of St. Joseph Health System, Orange, CA.

7

Case Consultation and Review: Matching Skills and Expectations

Given the nature of medical practice and the hospitals that institutionalize much of its values, it is not surprising that case consultation[1] plays a major role in the vitality and success of most ethics committees. If ethics committees had emerged in an educational rather than a clinical setting, they would have a somewhat different self-understanding and measure of success. However, much of the importance of consultation in the hospital culture involves the professionalization and compartmentalization of health care and the consequent model of knowledge, wisdom, and authority that involves the consultation of experts.

In another sense, this emphasis on consultation parallels medicine's focus on curing disease rather than either preventing it or helping patients cope with what cannot be cured. Ethics committee case consultation places similar emphasis on *curing* ethical problems, whereas ethics committee education emphasizes *preventing* ethical problems. Because ethics committees model themselves, albeit unconsciously, on the acute care setting in which they usually exist, it is understandable that they seem to measure their effectiveness by their degree of consulting activity.

If asked to rank-order their interest in the three functions of ethics committees — case consultation, policy development, and education — committees would likely rank consultation as their unchallenged first choice, even though they might also say that education is their most important function.

To the extent that case review/consultation receives the most attention from committees, it deserves scrutiny. If ethics in health care is perceived as primarily an issue of individual dilemmas and their resolution (May we? May we not? Should we? Must we?) and ethics committees are perceived as effective mechanisms for resolving these individual dilemmas, case consultation becomes the activity par excellence of the ethics committee.

However, the more broadly the goals of the committee are defined, the less evident it is that consultation deserves such a role. For example, the goals of the ethics committee might be defined in the following way: to enable the hospital community to perceive ethical issues; to promote practices and behaviors that correspond to good ethics; and to resolve current ethical conflicts and prevent future ones. The importance of case consultation in such a broad picture is substantially diminished other than as an occasion to educate staff. Educational activity and systemic change, such as policy development, will be predictably more effective than individual case consultation in reaching these broader goals.

Nevertheless, case review is likely to continue to be an important and highly visible committee activity. Recent proposed legislation in both New York and California uses multidisciplinary committees such as ethics committees to review various kinds of treatment decisions, such as those for incompetent patients without surrogates.[2] Such policy proposals imply that ethics committees are expected to be able to carry out case review in a competent and conscientious manner. Even if, conceptually, it is not the most important function of the committee, committees must take it very seriously.

Regardless of how committees feel or should feel about case consultation, it was certainly seen as the unique contribution of ethics committees by commentators who wrote in the early years.[3] It was also seen as the ethics committee's most problematic activity. It was feared that, frustrated with the kinds of decisions that were being made, some health care professionals as well as some ethicists might be overly anxious to become involved and do a better job. Critics of prospective case review by ethics committees feared that physicians would have their decision-making authority superseded and that a multidisciplinary group, many and perhaps most of which did not comprise physicians, would in effect end up practicing medicine.[4] Committees regularly promised themselves — and their members — that they were there only to recommend options or provide a forum for exploring the issues. But physicians, nurses, and others (including patients and their families) who asked for committee assistance frequently thought they were being told what to do or were being promised what would be done. Because committees are made up largely of health care professionals who are used to *acting* in such individual cases, many mixed messages may have been sent about what the committee can and will do and, in fact, what it does in the course of case review.

Models of Prospective Case Review

There are three general models for case review: medical, legal, and educational. How individuals and individual committees understand the concept of case review determines the kinds of procedures and protocols that are developed and, indeed, whether any procedures or protocols are in fact developed.[5]

The Medical Model

If committees understand themselves to be conducting something akin to a medical consultation, they are usually comfortable having one or two committee members (usually physicians, perhaps accompanied by a nurse or a chaplain) discuss the case with the health care team or the physician responsible for the patient's care. The medical model emphasizes *expertise* in clinical matters and ethical issues, and operates like an individual clinical ethicist. Expertise and authority are the hallmarks of this model and the original emphasis on multidisciplinary perspectives is much diminished, if not entirely eliminated. The medical model is very active and responsive, usually assuming that the patient will be visited (and perhaps even examined[6]) and that individuals involved in the case will be personally interviewed.[7] One health maintenance organization (HMO) hospital ethics committee that operates within the medical model has entertained the possibility of appointing its own consultants to examine the patient.

In the medical model of consultation, the ethics committee sees itself as a facilitator and instigator of new action or direction on the case in order to find resolution. It goes out to the case; the case does not come to it. The success of such consultation is seen in terms of the conflicts in the individual case being satisfactorily resolved and the patient's care proceeding along lines that are acknowledged by the ethics committee to be "ethically appropriate." Follow-up is usually conducted to ensure that matters have held together and progress has occurred. The attending physician is very likely to feel that he or she must justify a decision to act in ways other than those the committee has recommended.

The Legal Model

The legal model of consultation is based on thinking of case review as a type of legal hearing. Such review is likely to involve a larger number of people from the ethics committee (perhaps the whole committee) and the thorough hearing of "evidence" from all parties. Committees using a legal model are more likely to be concerned about whether patient or surrogate consent is obtained for conducting the review or whether notice is formally given to the patient/surrogate. There is likely to be greater attention paid to issues of due process.

Individuals asked to contribute information may feel as if they are undergoing cross-examination when they come before the committee. The committee may liken its role to that of a judge or jury asked to resolve a conflict between parties having different views on the correct way to proceed.

In this model, specific decisions or recommendations are common and members may even vote on the appropriate course of action from an ethical perspective. Such a view presumes a clear understanding of a standard for making these decisions and, as a result, a legal model often fits best with cases involving forgoing treatment in circumstances that courts have previously addressed and provided such a standard. Legally modeled case reviews often seem to resemble deciding what is *legally* possible, rather than what is *ethically* appropriate or permissible. Using a legal format may make dominance of legal (rather than ethical) factors inevitable, but law and ethics are peculiarly intertwined in some areas of bioethics. Appointing an individual to act as the patient's advocate (which implies that others are not advocates for the patient) emphasizes the assumption of adversarial stances in this kind of review. As the medical model assumes there is an expert who knows what should be done and can arrange for it to happen, so the legal model assumes that the dispute involves two (and only two) sides, each with something to be said for its view, and requires an individual or group to decide which side has the better arguments and therefore "wins."

The Educational Model

The educational model suggests a kind of egalitarian perspective that we are all in this together and can benefit from helping each other think about the issues. Such a model is often used by those who think of themselves as, and often call themselves, an ethics forum rather than an ethics committee. In this model, the group is committed to providing an opportunity for people to talk through patient care issues with a supportive group that understands the nature of the practical issues. It is not a forum for health care professionals alone but, rather, is as appropriate for a patient (or a patient's family) who does not know what to do as it is for a physician or nurse who does not know what to do.

The educational model downplays characterizing cases as conflicts (emphasized in the legal model) and emphasizes the importance of "multidisciplinarity" (minimized in the medical model). This model may not direct itself toward a specific case that will have a specific resolution but, rather, toward exploring the ethical dimensions of a situation. In such circumstances, it may be less critical than in the other models that the physician responsible for the individual case be involved (although it is always desirable to have the physician present, not least because of power imbalances and their relationship to problem resolution).

It is also less critical that the committee follow up on the specific case or provide any recommendations or preferred options, because the committee's job is to stimulate thoughtful discussion rather than to give permissions. The assumption in this model is that problems can be resolved if individuals of goodwill sit together and communicate their different perceptions, knowledge, intuitions, and thoughts. Emphasis is placed on process, active listening, and careful articulation of the issues. Out of this sharing context, a broader understanding of the problem will emerge, leaving the person who first had the question better able to resolve or cope with the situation. In this model, there is less emphasis on ethics per se than on clarifying communication and exploring perceptions. For example, when a nurse says that she is unwilling to participate in withholding artificial nutrition and hydration from a patient because to do so would be to kill the patient, a medical model consultation might focus on having the nurse understand that, in this case, feeding harms the patient or at least provides no benefit; whereas a legal model consultation might explain to the nurse that the patient is entitled to refuse treatment or that the courts have said this action is no different from stopping a ventilator. In a counseling/educational model consultation, the nurse is more likely to be asked to talk about the source of her feelings.

A hospital committee that has consciously chosen the educational model might describe its process in this way:

Our committee has opted for the educational model of case review in an attempt to promote broader discussion and involvement of all who sit on the case review subcommittee. The legal model was not chosen because it has been deemed to be too confrontational or adversarial. The medical model was not chosen for fear that the physician will feel compelled to follow the committee's recommendations and the committee will feel compelled to make a specific recommendation. Instead, our committee operates on the following basis—making the many individuals involved in the problem aware of the ethical and moral issues, clarifying the medical problem (if there has been miscommunication), discussing the ethical issues of concern and the ethical principles involved, defining the ethical dilemma, and then offering a variety of options to the physician or the patient (or surrogate) so that those individuals can decide how the problem should be settled. To maximize education, the case is then summarized and discussed with the entire committee, which often leads to discussion of other cases or other problems on the wards and in the clinics. Because the committee does not make specific recommendations, liability has not been an issue.

Committee Models and Review Requests

Each of these models has both strong and weak points; thus, a committee might use more than one model or one that is a hybrid of two or three. However, the ethics committee must be clear about which model it is using and make its perspective explicit to the inquiring physician or other person requesting consultation. Problems arise when there is a mismatch between the health professional who comes to the committee and the committee itself. If the physician is looking for a medical model consultation and the ethics committee uses a legal or educational model, everyone is likely to be dissatisfied. For example, one case that came to a committee involved an internist who was caring for an elderly woman in need of a surgical procedure to increase her comfort. Although the surgery was elective, her physician felt very strongly that the patient's quality of life would be greatly improved if she were to undergo the procedure. However, because the patient lacked decision-making capacity and had no family to act as a surrogate, the surgeon refused to perform the operation. The surgeon was concerned about legal consequences and agreed to do the procedure only if the ethics committee would agree that it was in the patient's best interest. The physician did not seek approval through the legal system because of the time that would be involved and the continued pain the patient would have to endure waiting for a legal decision. Therefore, the internist presented the issue to the committee as one of deciding what was in the patient's best interest. However, the entire discussion of the case proceeded along the lines of an educational model consultation in which the committee explored the issues of the patient's best interests. During the discussion, the physician sensed that the committee also felt that the patient should receive the procedure. However, at the conclusion of the meeting, when the physician asked whether the committee would make a note in the chart or formally state that it thought the surgery was in the patient's best interest, the committee responded that it did not make formal recommendations or chart notes and thus could not meet the physician's request, although the chairperson agreed that the surgery appeared to be in the patient's best interest. The physician left the meeting greatly irritated, convinced that ethics committees were moral wimps unwilling to act on their judgments.[8] In this case, the physician did not clearly state to the committee in advance what the physician wanted from it, nor did the committee explain what it was prepared to offer. If there had been greater clarity, it might have been possible for the committee to be of greater assistance to both patient and physician.

In another case, a physician told of a seriously ill patient who was found unconscious on the street; the patient had no known family. There was very little prospect of his gaining consciousness, but he was receiving maximal care in the intensive care unit. The attending physicians requested a nephrology consult, with a note stating that the patient would very probably soon lose renal function and need dialysis. The nephrologist examined the patient and wrote a note to the intensivists that the patient's prognosis was very poor and he was not sure that dialysis was appropriate. He was, however, convinced that the intensivists would insist on dialysis because otherwise the patient would die. When asked if he had considered going to the hospital's ethics committee about this case, he said: "Are you kidding? They'll just tell me to get social services to spend some more time trying to find some family member who can make the decision." This physician, too, wanted a specific kind of help. A committee that operated on a medical model might have helped him, but the legal model committee that existed in his hospital (which believed that its contribution was finished once it had determined who should make the decision) could not meet his needs.

Physicians are not the only ones who are often disenchanted by or suspicious of ethics committees. A newspaper story recounted the experiences of one family with a seriously ill newborn. When the ethics committee meeting was arranged, the child's grandmother believed that the baby would have his "day in court" at last and that the committee would surely agree to stopping treatment. At the end, the committee agreed that treatment was indicated, and the family felt they had not been adequately represented.[9] Similarly, a nurse described her experience in an ethics committee review involving a seriously ill newborn. In this instance, the committee voted to stop treatment. The nurse described herself as "shocked" and unprepared for her experience as well as for the ethics committee's "casualness" and lack of knowledge, suggesting that she had expected something more along the lines of an expert medical consultation.[10]

This is not meant to suggest that committees should give physicians or others who consult them whatever they want. However, it is meant to suggest that there are very different ideas about what an ethics committee does in its case consultation function and that if the committee fails, first, to understand clearly what it is prepared to offer and, second, to explain clearly to the physician or other inquirer in advance what is possible, the consultation experience may well be unsatisfying for everyone.

Nor, as previously mentioned, is this meant to suggest that committees can or should pursue only one model, although many do. Rather, these models respond to different needs and ethics committees need to think about what needs they are prepared to meet in their facility. Some committees conduct an educational model consultation in a case that seems to need that, but are willing to be much more directive in other cases where it seems appropriate. However, even if it is capable of moving from one model to another, the committee should be clear about what it plans to do in a particular case. For example, when nurses came to a committee asking for help in a specific case in which a physician had refused to write a DNR order for a terminally ill and competent patient who had requested that one be written, the committee (which could have and had previously responded in a very direct and interventionist manner) instead decided to engage in educational strategies for an entire department, feeling that the problem was more systemic than individual. The nurses, however, were left feeling that their immediate concerns were beyond the committee's skills or interests and, when the physician–patient relationship in the case continued to deteriorate, chose not to ask the ethics committee for further assistance.

John Fletcher and Phillip Eulie have observed that the clinical ethicist, accustomed to trying to facilitate smoother relationships among patients, families, and members of the health care team, often fails to see that in a medical-style consultation the consultant himself or herself becomes one of the players and falls into the same problematic relationships.[11] This can be equally true of committees. Committees ought to consider having someone with a good understanding of group process and individual psychodynamics (for example, social workers, psychiatrists, or psychologists) observe their case review process in order to be sure the committee is doing what it intends to be doing. In the midst of these frequently dramatic situations, the referees (and that is how committees often see themselves) often become players but still want to cite and to enforce the rules. Fletcher suggests that, in a particularly difficult case, he would have benefited from a psychiatric consult, which could have helped him understand the dynamics of the relationships that had developed in the course of the consultation process (particularly his own anger at the patient's family)—relationships he believed interfered with the resolution of the conflict. Such a consultation would have provided him (or an ethics committee) with a better understanding of his own involvement and would have led to a better process and outcome.

Forms of Consultation/Case Review

Regardless of which model or combination of models the committee adopts, the consultation must take some form and should involve a protocol. Case review can take at least four different forms: review by the committee as a whole, review by a consultation team, review by a care team, and review by a clinical ethics consultant, sometimes referred to as a "beeper ethicist." These forms are not mutually exclusive, and often the same institution will use a variety of these approaches depending on the circumstances. Each form has its strengths and weaknesses.

Whole Committee Review

Review by the committee as a whole is the most common form of case review, especially in committees that are just beginning to do case review. Even older, more experienced committees often use whole committee review for cases that seem particularly appropriate to that form (usually cases that do not need to be dealt with quickly and thus can wait until a meeting can be arranged). Whole committee review gives all members a chance to engage in ethical reflection in the context of actual decision making (even if they do not make the decision). When done well, this kind of review usually gives members a sense of accomplishment and community. It also can provide motivation for further reading and study. It is most likely to be done well if one person is designated to facilitate the discussion, initially explaining to everyone what is to be done and the order in which it is to be done.

Large group facilitators face significant challenges. They must create an atmosphere of trust in which the parties can express their positions and underlying interest, in which the parties and other participants in the group feel they have been heard and understood and *are* indeed heard and understood, and in which participants are able to explore options for resolution within the framework of the interests and views expressed by all the participants. In mediation, the facilitator is usually seen as a person who is neutral about the case at hand. In the ethics committee context, that is not usually the case, but the designated ethics committee facilitator should try to be so to the extent possible, leaving it to his or her colleagues on the committee to make contributions on the substance of the issue at hand.[12] The facilitator must have spent considerable time gaining a thorough knowledge of the case background information so that there are no sudden surprises. He or she must also be willing to control the discussion, making on-the-spot decisions about when a particular issue has been discussed sufficiently, when further discussion must be provoked, when it is time to move to the next item on the agenda, and so forth. In addition, the facilitator must be able to regularly summarize what has happened in the case review so far and to direct the participants to their next task. Without this leadership, there will be no clear sense of movement in the discussion.

The role of facilitator is crucial for any kind of case review but is particularly difficult in whole committee review, where there are likely to be many people present with different agendas (committee members and noncommittee members), different levels of understanding, and different abilities to articulate perspectives. People who have undertaken this role without fully understanding the facts of the case or carefully planning the case review can tell horror stories of consultations that left physicians or nurses feeling that *helpful* was the last word they would use to describe what they had just been through, or that left ethics committee members wondering what had just happened or family members feeling abused and abandoned.

Several steps need to be taken to minimize the chance of enduring this kind of debacle. First, the committee needs to develop a very structured protocol as to how the consultation is to proceed. Although a protocol may seem unnecessarily mechanical or rigid to many (after all, we are all friends and colleagues), it permits a level of control that may be necessary to prevent injured feelings, disorderly discussions, and undue polarization of views. (See the later section on case review protocols for a more detailed discussion.)

Second, the committee needs to select its facilitator very carefully. Some committees automatically give this role to the chairperson (who may or may not have any of the skills necessary); other committees, either in a fit of democracy or an attempt to distribute the burden, give everyone a chance to take on the facilitator role, despite the fact that many members will not have the skills to do it. It is unwise to use the role of facilitator in the whole committee prospective case review as a way to help people develop such skills. If they already have the skills, they can refine and improve them by taking on the responsibility of facilitation. But if they do not have the requisite skills, they should not try to learn them that way. The handling of case review is too important to both those who have brought cases to the committee and the committee's reputation to be handled in other than the best possible way.

Core Consultation Team Review

Many committees have concluded that whole committee review is too cumbersome a process to be used for all consultation requests. Thus, many committees set up a *core consultation team* consisting of a small number of committee members, sometimes including former committee members. Core committee members are usually more seasoned and experienced and often have already demonstrated their skills (both interpersonal and substantive) and interest in doing case review. This smaller group can provide a high level of competence in a more tightly defined system. The core team approach has many advantages. The committee can designate its strongest members to represent it in a context that can have enormous impact on the committee's credibility and status in the institution. A core committee review is also much more flexible and less intimidating than a whole committee review. Additionally, a core team that works together over time can develop a strong group identity.

However, there are also drawbacks, in many instances including a lost emphasis on multidisciplinarity (such consultation teams are sometimes composed primarily of physicians), as well as the loss of committee unity that is achieved through whole committee case review. Swenson and Miller believe that a core team is essentially a compromise position between whole committee review and individual consultant review.[13] If a committee chooses to use a core case review team, it should develop a procedure by which multidisciplinary representation on the team is maintained. Even then, however, there is the potential for core consultation teams to create a subtle hierarchy of expert and nonexpert members, which can have weakening effects on motivation and identity for the committee.

Some committees opt for small consultation teams because they believe the hospital is better served by ensuring that case review is provided in the clinical setting by individuals with the appropriate skills, knowledge, interest, and work flexibility that enables them to meet on short notice. However, the emphasis on work flexibility may bar some members (staff nurses, in particular) who otherwise would be desirable and even critical members of such a team. Before moving to a consultation team as an exclusive form of case review, the ethics committee should consider carefully what it is losing by this choice.

Committees should also be attentive to potential long-term problems with a core team, particularly the practice of informal consultation. Once a core group begins to work effectively, there is considerable probability that individual members of the core team, well educated and experienced in the process, will begin to conduct individual case reviews. This does not arise from arrogance or willful disregard for committee procedures. Rather, because the creation of the core group usually results from efficiency concerns in the context of an adequate sense of community trust, the individual core consultation team member may conclude that the response to a case is obvious, that it is foolishly time-consuming to meet with two or three colleagues to rehearse the obvious, and that her or his colleagues trust the individual enough to handle this case alone. All of this may be true; but at that point is the person acting as a representative of the ethics committee or as an individual health care professional who happens to be experienced in and knowledgeable about bioethics issues? Is this person speaking for the ethics committee or for himself or herself? A case review protocol should address the issue of informal review, ensuring that those doing case consultation clarify for themselves and others whether they are speaking for themselves as knowledgeable individuals or as members and representatives of the ethics committee using the committee's process.

Health Care Team Educational Review

Some ethics committees refuse to do case consultations in principle, even though they believe case consultations have a place in helping health care team members resolve their ethical problems. These committees see the actual team of caregivers as the appropriate community of ethical reflection for a given case. They judge that their providing case review would contradict this fundamental ethical conviction. These ethics committees see themselves as having a consultation role that is essential but indirect. Their responsibility is to educate the institution's care providers so that they are then able to do case consultations efficiently and comprehensively by and for themselves. Committees that limit their role to providing education must be sure that they provide it publicly and frequently. Using retrospective case review as a regular feature in grand rounds, brown-bag lunches, and in-service presentations will help the health care team to learn better how to address ethical issues only if these presentations also address communication problems and the institutional structures that create problems.

The problems with this model include the risk that staff and physicians will feel that the committee is unwilling to take any responsibility when it comes to real problems. The pressure to have the committee actually take on case review may be considerable as people become more aware that the institution has an ethics committee. For example, in one hospital in which the committee did not do case review, physicians, nurses, and administrators would call the committee chairperson and, after being told the committee did not do case review, would ask the chairperson for his or her personal thoughts. He would then informally offer them advice. Subsequently, there would be reports that "The ethics committee says we can do X." If the committee does not do case review, it should avoid this kind of ambiguous practice. The committee should prepare a list of resources (human and written) for those who request specific assistance.

Clinical Ethicist Review

Some institutions have individuals with special training in bioethics who are available for case consultation whenever they are needed. However, they may or may not work with the ethics committee in the course of consultation. Some commentators have suggested that clinical ethicists should do the consultations and the ethics committee should focus on policy review and writing and on more general education.[14] These clinical ethicists have training in a variety of fields, usually at the doctoral level. Some clinical ethicists are health care professionals (nurses, social workers, or physicians) with special training in ethics; others come from philosophy, theology, or other humanities fields, or from law or behavioral science, and acquire competence in clinical issues through study and direct experience of hospital life. (See chapter 10 for a more extensive discussion of ethics committees and clinical ethicists.)

A clinical ethics consultant can provide timely, efficient, and consistent responses to ethical problems in patient care. The consultant can get to know many professionals personally. Health care professionals, familiar with requesting consultations from medical specialists, probably are more likely to ask for help from an ethics consultant than from an ethics committee. Thus, if having more consultations is the goal of the ethics committee or of the institution, a clinical ethicist may be the best response. However, there are significant drawbacks to this response. A major problem with this form of case review is that no matter how competent the individual clinical ethicist may be, he or she remains one individual with all the limits that this brings: how the question will be framed, what vocabulary will be offered, how prescriptive the approach will be, how broad will be the range of ethically acceptable options offered, how familiar the individual is with all the institutional cultures involved, how personally approachable or likable this individual is, and so forth.

Involvement of the ethical community (if only symbolically by some representatives of that community) within the hospital is lost, as is any possibility of multidisciplinarity. This model also has the disadvantage of reinforcing the idea that ethics is like neurology or some other medical specialty—a field of technical expertise best carried out by highly trained professionals in intimate consultations. There are serious reasons to reject this parallel and its reinforcement in the minds of staff and patients, not the least being that it suggests that others in the health care facility have no ethical obligations to attend to.[15] If the health care system is to fully manifest its commitment to compassion and concern for patients and their families, as well as respect for the humanity of each individual, it must not convey the message that ethics belongs exclusively to "ethics experts" and that ethical issues exist only in certain kinds of cases where there are disagreements about what is the appropriate treatment decision or who is the appropriate decision maker.

Selection of the Preferable Form of Case Review

Given the different forms and models of conducting case consultation, how is a committee to decide what to use? Certainly there is no single best way. All these forms have proven consistently effective in the hands of some committees and all have been valuable in certain situations. However, there are reasons for preferring certain approaches over others as a routine way to do case review.

We assume that human dignity stands at the heart of ethical concern. Therefore, ethical issues—unlike orthopedic or neurological issues—are significantly present wherever human dignity is substantively at stake. We also presume that being conscious of, and responsive to, ethical reality is primarily an issue of fundamental humanity, not a professional skill belonging only to some educated people. Given these assumptions, the preferable forms of case review would be those that enable the largest number of people to increase their awareness of ethical reality and their ability to resolve its dilemmas, and those that demonstrate that ethical responsibility is a universal human calling, not a professional vocation. A form that enlarges case consultation rather than narrows it is preferable, though it should never be made so large that the dignity of the patients, their families, and the health care team is placed at risk.

Decisions about what form of consultation to use should not be based solely on efficiency concerns or on an administrator's comfort level with a particular individual or a group of individuals. It is clear that core consultation teams and clinical ethics consultants are more efficient ways to address these issues if the only thing that is desired is a reasonably rapid and competent resolution. And certainly some cases demand and deserve rapid resolution. But overall, ethics committees and institutions must think about the consultation function in as broad a form as possible. There will almost always be some individuals on a committee who are more skillful in interpersonal dynamics or ethical theory, and if the consultation function is to be narrowed, those individuals should be included and probably will be leaders. But to the extent that we are thereby saying "These are the people who know ethics," we will have lost the conceptual foundations of ethics committees themselves, which promised that all of us together were ethically stronger than any of us separately.

Case Review Protocols

Ethics committees that have been doing case consultation without a protocol and without problems may well say: "Why do we need it? We are doing just fine without it. We settle each new problem as it comes up." It is certainly true that committees can proceed in that way, but this approach does not necessarily instill confidence in those who come to the committee and see that the committee is not sure how to proceed in a somewhat novel situation and has to work out its rules on the spot. For example, the committee is asked to review a concurrent case in which it becomes quite clear that a physician (who is not present at the review) is in direct and conscious violation of a long-standing hospital policy (and, in essence, is violating the patient's legal rights) and seems to have no intention of changing his actions. The physician declined an invitation to attend the review, but the nurses involved in the case are present. This is no time to have to decide whether one of the committee's options is to report physicians who are violating policy and law to the medical executive staff.

There are arguments for and against such decisions, and the committee should have thought these out beforehand.

Similarly, a committee is in the process of a preliminary case consultation and the nurse (or a resident in a teaching hospital) says, "You won't let anyone know that I'm the one who told you about this case, will you?" It will do little to instill confidence in that person if the core team members say, "Oh, I don't know. We've never had a case like this before."

Protocols involve simple issues (the order in which the aspects of the case are discussed), complicated issues (whether a case consultation can begin without first informing the attending physician), and conventional ones (determining who can bring a case to the committee). Committees should be prepared to spend at least one full meeting considering these issues and portions of several more meetings considering the work of a subcommittee that is preparing specific documents. Protocols may involve separate guidelines and procedures for requesting and conducting a consultation, and forms for summarizing, reporting, and evaluating the consultation. The ethics committee at Foothill Hospital (Calgary, Alberta, Canada) includes guidelines and procedures for committee members who wish to publish work based on their consultations (the only such document we have seen that considers this).[16]

Consultation can be considered to be a three-stage process—intake, case review, and evaluation. A protocol should be developed for each stage.

The Intake Stage

In the intake stage of the consultation, the committee should diagnose the problem and determine the most effective way to address it. Many hospital chaplains, in particular, who are members of ethics committees deal with issues at this stage, often going back and forth between the individuals in conflict without involving the committee or even the core team. (Is this an informal ethics committee consultation, or an ethics consultation by a hospital chaplain? That question should be resolved by the intake protocol.) The intake process sets the stage for what follows and must be carefully considered.

Because intake is critical, it may not be wise to designate anyone and everyone on the committee to conduct this initial evaluation of the case. However, deciding who *will* do it is another critical part of this protocol. It is not necessarily appropriate (though it appears to be a common practice) to automatically delegate this responsibility to the committee chairperson. The questions listed in figure 7-1 should assist the committee in developing a protocol for this phase.

Figure 7-1. Proposed Intake Protocol Questions

1. Who may request a review from this committee?
2. Will the committee accept anonymous requests or provide anonymity?
3. Who on the committee should receive consultation requests?
4. What do committee members do when they receive such calls?
5. From whom is information gathered?
6. Who gathers that information, and how?
7. Is the patient or family informed that a review has been requested?
8. Is patient or family permission requested to conduct a review?
9. Are patients or families asked to attend? Can they request attendance?
10. How does the committee decide whether to review this case?
11. If the committee is unable or unwilling to review this case, what will the requester be told?
12. Where is the consultation held?
13. Who is asked to attend the review?
14. Does everyone meet at the same time?
15. Is informed consent given to those who requested the review? (That is, do they know what to expect? Who tells them, and how?)
16. How does the committee ensure that information is accurate and complete?

The Case Review Stage

The protocol for the case review discussion involves the following:

- Determining the meeting place and time (with all the attendant psychological messages sent by that decision)
- Making introductions
- Reminding members of confidentiality requirements
- Explaining the process
- Structuring and announcing the order of elements in the discussion, for example:
  - Factual matters first, with assessment that all necessary medical and other factual information is available or can be obtained
  - Preferences of patients, surrogates, and health care team members and reasons for those preferences
  - Ethical values at stake in various courses
  - Identification of options
- Concluding the discussion, with summary and explanation of what is to happen next (if anything)

Figure 7-2 is a list of questions that should help the committee work through this stage of the process and develop the appropriate protocols.

The Postreview and Evaluation Stage

The third stage includes specifying the kind of records to be kept, where they are to be kept, and who is to keep them, as well as what information about the review is to be provided to others and who these others are. Evaluation of case reviews can be conducted with both those involved in the process outside the committee and those involved within the committee itself. The committee may want to prepare specific evaluation forms for each of these groups, or it may want its evaluations to be more general. The questions provided in figure 7-3 should be considered in designing the protocol for this stage of the process.

A committee that has thought through and developed three such protocols is in a better position to explain what it does in case review—to itself, to new members, to the institution, and to those who seek consultation assistance from it. Development and implementation of these protocols also helps the committee to ensure that it does in fact do what it says it will do. Documentation of the process and of each individual case consultation may seem time-consuming, but it addresses both the issue of the committee's accountability for its authority (as limited as that authority may seem to be) and concerns about liability. There is only one reported case of a hospital ethics committee having been sued (the *Bouvia* case, in California, in 1986), and it was subsequently dropped. However, as in any situation in

Figure 7-2. Proposed Case Review Protocol Questions

1. Who facilitates the meeting and how is that decision made?
2. How does the facilitator get background information on the case?
3. Where is the meeting held? (Does the committee go to the requester, or does the requester come to the committee?)
4. How are arrivals at the meeting scheduled? (Everyone at once? Staggered?)
5. What are the committee's goals with respect to case review?
6. What are those present told about confidentiality, review purpose and potential outcomes, structure of the meeting, time limits?
7. Who comes to resolution on the problem, the committee or the caregivers/patient?
8. Does someone keep notes during the meeting?
9. What kind of records are kept of the meeting?
10. Will the committee write a chart note on request? Without request? Despite the physician's request that no chart note be written?

Figure 7-3. Proposed Postreview Evaluation Protocol Questions

1. If this is not whole committee review, how is the larger committee apprised of it?
2. What follow-up is conducted with respect to the case?
3. Does follow-up depend on the committee's preferences or those of the caregivers or patient?
4. What kind of evaluation is conducted? What are the purposes of evaluation?
5. Does the committee have a format for self-evaluation?
6. Who receives case summaries and who receives case evaluations?
7. Is there anything the committee will not do with respect to consultation?

which the threat of litigation exists, good documentation of the process and outcome, showing prudence and good ethical judgment, is the best defense against any allegations of impropriety or misconduct.[17]

Documentation

Committees need to document the consultation process, but also must consider both the kind and degree of documentation. At a minimum, decisions should be made about records of the consultation process (including subsequent evaluations or follow-up), and chart notes.

Case Consultation Records

There are two views on keeping records, deriving mostly from the difference between the case review models. If case review is to be like a medical consultation or a legal review, there will be a commitment to thorough record keeping. In this view, case consultations (regardless of the form used) should be thoroughly documented in a consistent manner, not only for legal purposes but also for research purposes. Such committees often have developed forms to record each case review summary in the same format, and they keep their records in locked cabinets to ensure confidentiality. If a committee is asked to prepare a report describing its case review practices over the previous three years, such documentation should provide good data for a prompt reply. This view assumes that the committee has a high level of accountability for its practices.

For committees that understand case review to be a more open-textured activity, such as counseling or education, the justification for keeping detailed records seems more obscure. Such committees are likely to keep more general records, for example, committee minutes. There is often resistance to more detailed record keeping because the purpose of this activity is not clear. The kind of record this model requires is sometimes no more than a description of the case itself, which can be used in other educational forums.

As a practical matter, however, the committee should discuss this issue with its superiors. For example, what kind of records does the administration, medical staff executive committee, or board of trustees expect it to keep? Such a discussion should involve an understanding of the purpose of the records. Failing to keep records or keeping sketchy records so that no records will be available to the court in the case of litigation is poor justification for a decision to minimize record keeping. If litigation arises, good records are the committee's best defense. An additional consideration is that if case consultation is to become a more dominant role for committees, it will help to have good documentation for purposes of evaluation.

Chart Notes

Many committees still remain uncertain as to whether they should write in the chart, and there seems to be fairly even division between those who do and those who do not. A chart note is always appropriate if the committee thinks it has been directly involved in patient care decisions, but it is not always necessary. However, if the committee is asked to document its involvement by the physician or nurse involved in the case, the committee should ask itself very seriously why it would *not* respond positively to such a request. That is, if the committee has made recommendations or indicated that one or more options would be ethically appropriate, it should be willing to record that that is what it did. On the other hand, if the committee has done nothing more than discuss some general principles or similar cases that have been analyzed in various ways, it is not clear why the health care professional would want the committee to document that in the chart.

Presumably the committee has written its own case summaries. If the committee wishes to take the blanket position never to make chart notes, a compromise position would be to provide the physician promptly with a copy of the committee's summary of its discussion and permit him or her to include this in the medical record under his or her own authority. Ultimately, a committee that fails to document its case review has misunderstood its role, which is not to make decision processes more secretive but to make them more open. A refusal to document leads to fear and suspicion about what really goes on at an ethics committee consultation session.

Patient Access to the Consultation Process

Case consultation is such a sensitive issue that, in the early years, many committees accepted review of cases only from physicians. Although this has political justification, its moral justification is hard to understand. As case review has become more accepted by physicians, committees have found it possible to make themselves available to anyone involved in a situation who believes there is a serious ethical problem.

Requests for Committee Help

Although a few committees continue to restrict access to physicians, most are willing, at least in principle, to consider cases at the request of the patient or the patient's family. However, as a matter of practice, that seldom happens. It would certainly be peculiar if a committee created to ensure that patient interests were protected was unwilling to accept requests from patients or their families. It is apparently not peculiar, however, that clinical ethicists, for political reasons, are often unwilling to accept a consultation request from anyone other than the patient's attending physician. The basis for this judgment appears to be that they will never get any requests if they become involved at the clinical level without the attending physician's permission; that is, that they will be perceived as interfering. The same concern might be expressed by ethics committees.

It is probable that few patients or their families come directly to the committee for consultation, either because it is arranged by their nurse or patient representative or because they are unaware that an ethics committee exists in the hospital or that it is open to them. In the past few years, many committees have written patient brochures on forgoing treatment policies. These brochures often describe something about the committee's availability to the patient in case of decision problems, and may lead to patients' (or their families') seeking out the committee's help. In addition, the Patient Self-Determination Act has spurred institutions to inform patients of the fact that there is an ethics committee in the hospital and that it can help them.

Consent or Notice for Case Review

The question of whether patients should be asked to give informed consent to, or be notified of, an impending ethics committee case review continues to be a matter of dispute in the literature.[18] In practice, patients (and their families) are seldom either given notice or asked formally for consent. They may be asked if they would like to have the ethics committee discuss the case (a practice that seems to be more than notice but less than consent). Or, a nurse may suggest to the patient and/or family that he or she would like to talk with the ethics committee about the situation (something like notice but nothing like consent). In cases involving a physician or a nurse who is uncertain about specific treatment questions (Would it be all right to recommend stopping the ventilator? Am I required to participate in dialyzing this patient?), there is no reason to involve the patient or family. Here, the caregiver appears to be inquiring about his or her own professional responsibilities. But often, even in cases that directly involve the patient's or family's views and preferences, there is neither notice nor consent.

Patients and/or families should be informed about the prospective consultation (except in cases where the physician is inquiring about his or her own professional rights and duties), should have the nature of the consultation process fully explained to them, and should be offered the opportunity to talk directly with the committee. This is not so much a matter of providing appropriate due process (as Susan Wolf has called for)[19,20] as it is one of providing *good* process (as Vicki Michel has called it).[21] The use of the phrase *due process* implies that this is essentially a legal proceeding. If case consultation results in ethics committees making decisions for patients or adjudicating between the preferences of caregivers and patients, due process protections would be more appropriate.

It is less a need for due process than that of respect for persons that leads to the presumption that patients and families be given notice about case review. When those gathering information for a case review talk to families or patients about their understanding and preferences, the patient or family should know why the information is being gathered. The committee should also make clear to them the possible outcomes of the review and its process. If you were a family member and disagreed with a physician about the kind of treatment to be given to your loved one, would you expect an ethics committee to side with you? If the committee did not, would you think that it had ganged up on you to protect the physician? The answer is probably yes to both these questions. That is why it is so important to ensure in advance that patients and their families understand why there is to be a case consultation and what the potential outcomes of the process are in this institution.

However, all issues that come to the committee are not so adversarial. Sometimes the adversarial aspect is between nurse and physician with respect to what the policy in the hospital is. For example, if a patient wishes a DNR order to be written and the physician refuses to write it but does not tell the patient this fact, should the patient be informed of the nurse's request that the ethics committee review this physician's action? It could be argued that the patient has made his or her position clear and that the issue is how to respond to the physician. Yet it might be that the patient's attachment to the physician is such that the patient would rather not have the DNR order than force the physician to do something he or she is unwilling to do. In such a case, the tendency of ethics committees might be to ensure that the patient's wishes are followed, that is, to get the DNR order written in one way or another without involving patient or family—a conclusion supported by most bioethics writing. But it is possible that in bypassing the patient, the committee has lost the opportunity to strengthen the relationship between patient and physician. If that were so, the committee could rightly be criticized for interfering in the physician's practice.

The matter of consent from or notice to patients and/or families is problematic in many cases and should be taken more seriously by committees. Perhaps the committees, grounded as they are in medical practice, see case review as a minor matter in the course of providing care, rather like a blood test, which it is free to conduct if the need for review is persuasive. It would certainly be ironic if the ethics committee were found to be practicing the same old paternalism that it was thought to be replacing.

Conclusion

Consultations seem to many to be the lifeblood of the ethics committee; yet apparently many committees are experiencing fewer requests for consultations (which may account for reported symptoms of anemia in the ethics committee world). This appears to be a relatively common experience in institutions where committees appeared to conduct quite competent and successful consultations as well as in those in which the quality might have been somewhat more uneven. The explanations posited for this circumstance have been that (1) staff no longer call on the committee because they have been dissatisfied with what the committee had to offer in previous circumstances; (2) staff are better able to handle these matters by themselves because of committee education or the attention given to bioethical issues on television, in the mass media, and at professional educational forums; and (3) staff have been frustrated by the committee's slow pace in handling cases and do not recognize the committee as the appropriate mechanism for their problems. Another explanation may be that the committee has helped the hospital community to better understand how to address some ethical issues, but has not helped it to recognize other issues about which there is less publicity. Other committees have not experienced a decline in the number of cases they are asked to review, but that number was never large.

Staff at some hospitals are reluctant to involve ethics committees because they do not want the committee to interfere. However, this attitude can change. For example, in one VA hospital the surgeons were extremely hostile to the ethics committee's "interference" with patients on the surgical ward. However, they were delighted to call on the committee to help intervene with a family who demanded more and more treatment, including surgery, for a patient who was already in extremis. The committee achieved credibility with the surgical staff when it helped resolve a dilemma from which the staff could see no route of escape. When staff reach such a level of frustration that their only recourse is the ethics committee, and the committee is able to respond in a way that leads to a release of that frustration, the committee may then be seen as a valuable resource. However, committees need to be careful about developing responses that seem to be intended to curry favor with physicians.

Staff at yet other hospitals may be reluctant to call on the ethics committee for consultation because they are not sure what they may be getting themselves in for. And, to the extent that few committees have formal consultation protocols, this attitude may be justified. Ethics committees cannot think that just because they are called *ethics* committees their competence, goodwill, effectiveness, and desirability are taken for granted. They must be prepared to give informed consent to those who come to them and to look at improving their consultation process. Regular reflection about the process can surely lead to improvement and greater acceptance in the hospital.

There are many reasons why a committee might not be asked to consult frequently. But the most probable general explanation is that ethics committees are relatively unknown in most hospitals, even when they have been in existence for five years or more. Staff and physicians do not know much about them and patients and their families are doubtless less aware. Mid-size and large health care institutions are places in which people on one floor often have little or no idea of what is going on next door or on the next floor. Surgical nurses often are unaware that the working conditions of nurses on the medical wards differ so greatly from their own. Pediatrics staff live in a different world from staff working with adult patients. Thus, ethics committees are not unique in their invisibility, and it is not surprising that they do relatively little case consultation, despite the length of their existence in the hospital. However, there are many other things to occupy their attention. And there is much that they can do to help increase the hospital community's awareness of their presence.

Exercises

1. Put yourself in the place of a family member who has just been involved in a case review with your committee. Would you see the committee (or the facility) as concerned about you or your family? What would be the evidence of that? What did that committee do to make sure you understood the process you were engaged in? Beforehand? During the review? What kind of closure was provided for you?

2. After the committee has conducted either a prospective or a retrospective review and only committee members are present, have each member suggest one thing that he or she wishes had been different during the review and one thing that the member was pleased occurred.

3. Have each member write down how he or she thinks multidisciplinarity on the committee made the case review better for the patient, the patient's family, and the health care team.

4. Complete the following sentence: Our ethics committee does case consultation but

_____.

The responses will tell you something about how committee members understand the process. For example, the response "Our ethics committee does case consultation but doesn't take cases from nurses" suggests that the writer believes that case consultation should involve taking cases from nurses. Thus, the "but" gives you some sense of how people understand the category and what follows is something that is unusual or unexpected.

5. Consider the following cases:
   A. A young man has asked to be a kidney donor for his older brother. The transplant center believes that some kind of financial promise has been made by the brother who needs the kidney, and the transplant physician is reluctant to accept the donor and seeks the advice of the committee. Should the committee inform the patient or his brother of the physician's request for case review?
   B. A physician seeks the committee's advice because he has an HIV-positive patient who is a nurse anesthetist. The physician wishes to discuss whether he has any responsibility to discuss the nurse's condition with the nurse's employers. Should the committee inform the patient of the physician's request?
   C. Two physicians disagree about whether a very expensive drug should be offered to patients. They have come to this question in the course of a particular case in which both have been involved. Physician A refused to provide the drug because she thought (1) it was unlikely to work and (2) it would pose significant risks to the patient, and instead recommended a surgical procedure. Subsequent to the surgery, physician B saw the patient and, in discussing the decision with physician A, requested consultation with the ethics committee to discuss whether the patient should have had the drug. Should the committee inform the patient of this request?
   D. A patient in a persistent vegetative state has an advance directive saying that he wants treatment stopped in this circumstance and naming his daughter as his agent in a durable power of attorney for health care. However, the daughter has asked the physician to continue treatment. The physician in turn seeks the advice of the committee. Should the committee inform the daughter of the physician's request?

6. Distribute parts for a role-play to members of the committee in advance of the meeting and conduct a mock case review just as you would a formal request. Encourage a candid discussion afterward of people's feelings about the process and the substance of the review. Make sure that people who are playing the roles reveal information about their character only as it would necessarily be revealed, and provide each character with adequate information about who they are and what they are doing. (Two sample role-play cases are included in appendix 7-1.)

Notes and References

1. We use the terms *case review* and *case consultation* interchangeably to describe this activity. Although the terms have rather different connotations, we prefer not to send a message that this activity is exactly like either a medical consultation or a legal review.

2. Miller, T., editor. *When Others Must Choose: Deciding for Patients without Capacity.* Albany, NY: Health Education Services, 1992; California Health and Safety Code Section 1418.8 (passed 1992).

3. See, for example, Cranford, R. E., and Doudera, A. E., editors. *Institutional Ethics Committees and Health Care Decision Making.* Ann Arbor, MI: Health Administration Press, 1984.

4. Ross, J. W. Ethics committees: a turn for the worse? *Mobius* 3(3):85–89, 1983.

5. Ross, J. W. Why cases sometimes go wrong. *Hastings Center Report* 19(1):22–23, 1989.

6. LaPuma, J., and Schiedermayer, D. L. Must the ethics consultant see the patient? *Journal of Clinical Ethics* 1(1):56–59, 1990.

7. Arguments rejecting a medical model with respect to the ethics committee seeing the patient are presented by Iserson, K., with the contrary view presented by Pruit, R. L. Should the ethics committee visit the patient? No, and yes. *HEC Forum* (3)1:19–26, 1991.

8. Ross, J. W. Informed consent for physicians: another consultation caveat. *Ethical Currents* 19:7,9, 1989.

9. Theroux, P. Family's painful choice over brain-damaged infant. *Los Angeles Times,* Dec. 15, 1988, Section 5A, p. 1ff.

10. Edwards, M. Decision by committee. *American Journal of Nursing* 86(7):796–97, July 1986.

11. Fletcher, J., and Eulie, P. Code him until he's brain dead. In: C. M. Culver, editor. *Ethics at the Bedside.* Hanover, NH: University Press of New England, 1990, pp. 8–28.

12. Gibson, J. M., and West, M. B. Facilitating medical ethics case review: what ethics committees can learn from mediation and facilitation techniques. *Cambridge Quarterly* 1(1):63–74, 1992.

13. Swenson, J. M., and Miller, R. B. Ethics case review in health care institutions: committees, consultants, or teams. *Archives of Internal Medicine* 152:694–97, 1992.

14. LaPuma, J., and Toulmin, S. E. Ethics consultants and ethics committees. *Archives of Internal Medicine* 149:1109–12, 1989.

15. Ross, J. W. Ethics consultation: the ethics committee or the ethics consultant? *HEC Forum* 2(5):289–98, 1989.

16. For commentary on this issue, see Riis, P., and Nylenna, M. Patients have a right to privacy and anonymity in medical publication: editorial. *Journal of the American Medical Association* 256(20):2720, 1991.

17. *Bouvia v. Superior Court, Glenchur, et al.,* (225 Cal Rptr., 297 [1986]).

18. For example, see, Stidham, G. L., Christensen, K. T., and Burke, G. F. The role of patients/family member in the hospital ethics committee's review and deliberation. *HEC Forum* 2(1):3–18, 1990; Veatch, R. M. Advice and consent. *Hastings Center Report* 19(1):20–22, 1989; and Wolf, S. M. Due process in ethics committee case review. *HEC Forum* 4(2):83–96, 1992.

19. Wolf, S. M. Ethics committees and due process: nesting rights in a community of caring. *Maryland Law Review* 50(3):798–858, 1991.

20. Wolf, S. M. Due process in ethics committee case review. *HEC Forum* 4(2):83–96, 1992.

21. Michel, V. Ethics committee procedure: due process or good process. *Ethical Currents* 30:6–7, 1992.

Appendix 7-1. Sample Role-Plays

Case 1: May This Patient Refuse Treatment?

An older female patient presents to the emergency department (ED) with severe abdominal pain. She has a fever and is hypotensive. She is given analgesics in the ED and decides that she is well enough to go home. The physician and a surgical consultant urge her to stay because the tests suggest she might have biliary sepsis, which would require close monitoring, antibiotics, and possibly surgical exploration. The patient absolutely refuses intensive therapeutics. Although the attending physician discusses the situation extensively with both the patient and her son, she still insists on going home (despite a systolic pressure of 70). The patient says she understands that the doctors think she is seriously ill and might die and that she does not want to die, but that she does not believe she is that sick. She finally agrees to stay but asks to discuss the situation with her son in private, after which she repeats her desire to go home, asserting that the pain is subsiding. Her son reports that she thinks the physicians are overly worried. (During a previous hospitalization for gallbladder removal, she had been in the ICU for three days because of complications and had repeatedly told her nurse how much she disliked being there.) When asked by the physician for his views, her son says that he wants his mother to live, but that he isn't about "to try to convince her of anything" and that if she wants to go home, it's all right with him.

The Roles

Mrs. Candela (the patient)   You are a 65-year-old woman who has been a widow for 15 years. (Your husband died of cancer.) You own your own small home and have not worked for the past 10 years because of a variety of medical problems, primarily stemming from your long history of diabetes mellitus. You live on a very small pension and, although money is tight, you are able to manage and control your own financial affairs. You had two children—Robert and Elena. Elena was killed in a traffic accident five years ago. Robert, the younger child, had a difficult adolescence and always got into trouble. He once served time in a juvenile facility for a minor offense, and you and he do not always get along. However, because of your poor health, you are grateful that he is there to take you places and to perform any kind of work for you that involves lifting or carrying. Although you love him, Robert is a worry to you because he is still so wild and sometimes rough. He drinks, and when he drinks he sometimes becomes very angry. Also, things sometimes disappear from around the house and you suspect that he has taken them and sold them, although he denies it. He doesn't have a job and doesn't seem to want one, preferring to live with you rent free and live off the little money you give him for helping you.

     You have had a lot of experience with physicians and healers (you always go to both when you are seriously ill, but just to healers for ordinary sickness). Six months ago, your gallbladder had to be removed, which required about two months of recuperation. Because of some minor complications, you had to stay in the ICU for several days. You couldn't sleep because of the lights and the noise, and you had no privacy at all. In fact, you think it probably took you so long to recover from surgery because of additional time in the ICU: it just made you sicker. Then, when you were almost back to normal, you broke your arm when you fell during an argument with Robert. And now you have this sharp pain in your stomach. It feels terrible, a lot like the pain you felt when you found out your mother had been killed in a bus accident—and that was about the worst pain you ever had. When you told Robert about the pain, he insisted that you go to the ED right away. You were reluctant to go because you thought the pain would go away if you waited it out as it was likely just nerves; if it didn't, you would at least consult your *curandero* before going to the hospital. When you have had sharp pains like this in the past, his medicine made you feel better pretty fast. But Robert insisted on bringing you to the ED. You don't want to stay in the hospital again. Besides, if you are in the hospital, Robert will get into trouble. Who knows what will happen if you are not home for days at a time?

*Robert Candela
(the patient's son)*

You are 25 years old and an unemployed high school dropout. When you were younger, you became involved with a gang and got into some trouble, which led to a brief incarceration in a juvenile facility. Although you pulled out of the gang a few years ago, you still have friends who are gang members. Sure, you drink a little, you do a little drugs, but nothing hard or dangerous—no coke or smack or PCP. Just a little marijuana now and then. Just like everybody else. You don't quite know what you're doing with your life, and you aren't interested in discussing your life with your mother or any doctors. Your mother is usually okay, but she sometimes drives you crazy because she's always after you to get a job, quit drinking, and stop seeing Fred or Max or whoever. Nothing you do seems to suit her. She's lucky you're willing to live with her and take care of her, given that she can't do anything for herself. She doesn't seem to realize that she'd be in a nursing home if it weren't for you. The way you see it, taking care of her is your job.

When your mother broke her arm, you and she were arguing about your staying out too late one night. You were plenty mad, okay, but that's not against the law. Just as you gestured strongly with your arm, your mother walked right into it. The impact knocked her into the table and broke her arm. So when you took her to the hospital that day, the docs were all over you suggesting you had broken her arm. They even threatened to report you for something called elder abuse. You sure didn't hit her, even if plenty of times you felt she deserved it. Well, you're not going to give them another chance to carry on about how you aren't taking care of your mother, or about how you're being mean to her. As soon as she started complaining about this pain, you took her right to the hospital so those doctors could figure out what to do.

And now they're asking *you* to figure out what to do! Boy, this is their problem and hers; they have to work it out, not you. Actually, you're not sure the doctor is right. She doesn't look sick, she did fine on a bunch of tests, and now she says the pain is getting better. She says she doesn't want to stay in the hospital and she wants you to tell them so. What's it to you? If she says she wants to go home, then she should get to go home. Doctors aren't the police, and a hospital isn't a prison.

Ms. Ames (the ED nurse)

You are one of the nurses currently assigned to the ED. As it happens, you took care of Mrs. Candela when she was in the ICU following her gallbladder operation. You remember her talking a lot about how she hated being in the ICU, how being there made her feel as if she were waiting to die, and how anybody sick enough to die ought to be able to be at home with the things and people they know. She also had some odd ideas about medicine and medical treatment, apparently based on what you would characterize as folk beliefs. She didn't appear to have any religious affiliation and she never wanted chaplains to visit; instead, she seemed to attribute healing power to certain artifacts. For example, she kept a little grey and reddish rock with her all the time. Misplacing that innocuous-looking stone would send her into a tizzy. And she always wanted to drink special teas, but her physician wouldn't let her have them. He told her that it would be better if she waited until she went home and then they'd provide her with strength, but in the hospital it was better to have just the hospital's medicines and teas.

You're not too fond of her son Robert. You don't think that Mrs. Candela is either, although she never said anything specific. You think she's a little afraid of him; he *is* really big and she's so small and fragile. Also, he seems very aggressive. He never asked for anything nicely—just made demands. He always acted as if she was the only patient in the hospital and he was the only family member visiting. His motto was: Do it right now! But, in spite of all this, you like Mrs. Candela a lot. You would hate to see her leave right now because she's really sick, but, on the other hand, she really hates the hospital. And she admits that she might have a serious illness, so if that's what she wants to do, maybe that's what she should do. If she gets worse, you think Robert would bring her back right away. Anyway, what can you do? Strap her down to a bed and put her in the ICU against her wishes? You don't want to be a part of that.

Dr. Wyatt (the attending physician)

Mrs. Candela is something of a mystery to you. On the one hand, she seems to understand everything; but on the other hand, she doesn't want to stay in the hospital and you think there's a significant chance that she may die or at least be in the ICU for even longer if she doesn't. She seems to be compliant, but when she gets an idea in her head, she doesn't appear to really hear anything you say. You are concerned about patients' rights to make their own decisions, but you don't think that this is what their rights are about. For example, you asked her if she wanted to die and she said no. So it's not that her quality of life is so terrible that she doesn't want to be treated, she just has this idea that she's not sick. But she's wrong. However, what's odd is that she's hypotensive but not dizzy or faint. You had her stand up to undergo the physical exam because you thought she would realize how terrible she felt and how sick she was, but she just took it in stride. You even did a repeat blood pressure reading using a cuff around her thigh because you thought that maybe the arm reading was wrong—but it wasn't. You don't know why she's standing up or even conscious right now.

You suspect that her son may be trying to talk her into something. She agreed that she needed treatment until she talked to him. Then, suddenly, she said she was feeling better. The pain has subsided because she's got all that analgesia in her, but in a few hours, it will wear off. If you can just keep her here talking, the pain will return and make her realize how sick she is. Your guess is the son told her something that made her want to leave—perhaps that we were after her money. That's what they all say nowadays. And he's the one who broke her arm. Maybe you should talk to her about him! You think that if you let her leave now, you would be the one guilty of elder abuse.

Case 2: Must This Patient Be Treated?

The patient suffered a stroke four months ago. He opened his eyes six weeks after the incident, but since then, he has been completely unresponsive. He remains on the ventilator and has been diagnosed by the neurologist as being in a persistent vegetative state. His wife insists that everything necessary to preserve his life be done for him—antibiotics, CPR, feeding, ventilator support, and so on. (She has also mentioned that if her husband's kidneys fail, she wants dialysis.) The only other involved family member is the patient's elderly mother, who is grieving and confused. She is allowing her daughter-in-law to make the decisions.

Several nurses caring for the patient, as well as the case management committee, have suggested strongly that he is not going to benefit from further treatment. Besides, his presence in the ICU is causing problems—he is using a bed that has often been needed for other patients; the nurses feel that treatment is both futile and an inappropriate use of resources, including their own time; and his wife is demanding and hostile whenever she visits, complaining loudly that the hospital is not doing all it can for her husband.

The Roles

The Neurologist	You feel strongly that continued treatment of this patient is medically and ethically inappropriate. You have been thinking and reading about the inequities in this country regarding access to health care. Millions of Americans do not have even basic care because they have no health insurance. Here is a perfect example of the problem with our system—a patient who cannot benefit from care is being treated at the cost of over $1,500 a day. The family should not have the right to insist on futile treatment. You have heard the hospital has an ethics committee, and you think the committee should review this case and recommend a solution.

You talk to Dr. Falvey, the chairperson of the committee, and tell him that if the ethics committee is worth anything to the medical staff and the hospital, it should tell the wife that the hospital will no longer treat her husband aggressively. Dr. Falvey tells you that the committee will review the case, but will not make a decision. (You tell him the committee is a wimp.) He also says that the wife must be given an opportunity to be present. Although you think it's a bad idea for her to be there, you agree to present the case. |
| *Chairperson of the Ethics Committee* | The neurologist has asked to present the case of a patient on a ventilator in the ICU. The case management committee, some of the nurses, and especially the neurologist believe that continued treatment is futile and should no longer be offered. However, the patient's wife is insisting on all possible treatment.

The neurologist wants to speak to you, ask the committee to recommend that treatment be discontinued. When you tell him that the committee does not make such decisions, he characterizes the committee as wimps, but wants to present the case anyway. You also tell him that the wife must be given an opportunity to be present to voice her concerns. Although he doesn't like this idea much either, he agrees. The neurologist, the attending physician, one of the nurses, and the wife will all be present at the ethics committee meeting. |
| *A Nurse from the ICU* | You are one of the nurses in the ICU caring for a man who has been on a ventilator for four months. The neurologist feels strongly that treatment is futile and should be discontinued, and the case management team, most of the other nurses, and the attending physician all agree.

The wife has alienated you and the other nurses by her demands and accusations. You appreciate her attachment to her husband, her difficulty in accepting that he has no prospect for recovery, but you think she needs to face reality. Nobody would want this kind of treatment for himself or herself. |
| *The Attending Physician* | You have attended the patient ever since he was admitted to the hospital four months ago. However, you do not know what kind of care he would |

have wanted, because you and he never discussed these matters. You are aware that shortly before the stroke, the wife learned that her husband had been having an affair with a coworker. She told you this, brokenheartedly, explaining that she never had a chance to understand what was happening. You think she needs professional help to adjust to her husband's situation. Treatment isn't hurting this patient, and if everyone could focus on the wife in a supportive way, you think it could work out.

The neurologist wants to take the case to the ethics committee and you reluctantly agree to go with him, uncomfortable with his aggressive approach, and wonder whether it is right to ace the wife out of the decisions.

Wife of Patient

You refuse to accept what the doctors are telling you—that your husband will never regain consciousness. He woke up six weeks after his stroke, and you believe he may recover if only the hospital would do its job. You think the hospital is just trying to get rid of you, and the doctors are afraid they will not be paid for his care. (He is covered by an HMO, which, as far as you know, will pay all his hospital and doctor bills.) You insist that your husband get whatever treatment is necessary, including dialysis in the event his kidneys fail.

Just before the stroke, you learned that your husband was having an affair with a coworker. You are angry, hurt, unfinished.

8

Evaluation and Self-Assessment: Determining How Much Ethics Committees Need to Do

It is evident that few ethics committees do much, if any, evaluation of their own work. Furthermore, virtually no systematic evaluation of ethics committees has been done by either hospitals or outside groups. Committees are reluctant to evaluate themselves and their work for many reasons. First, evaluation takes a great deal of time and energy, and there appears to be no external call for committees to do it. Most committees feel this time and energy could be better spent on "more fruitful" activities. Second, committees may be concerned that their work will be found inadequate or that individual members who do not "score" well enough will become estranged from the committee and discouraged from serving on it. Third, many committee members volunteer a lot of their time, often receiving little hospital support and no particular credit. Given that, ethics committee members may believe that their contribution need not be judged. Fourth, the people attracted to ethics committees quite often assume that if they are satisfied with what they are doing, that is good enough.

These are understandable reasons for committees not to rush to evaluation, particularly for the vast majority of committees that have been in existence for only a few years. Given that committees generally meet one to two hours a month (a very active committee might meet three to four hours a month), they cannot be expected to take on too much other work. Yet, if ethics committees are to be taken seriously in the future, they must take evaluation seriously. If they are to justify the commitment of institutional resources, the institution has a right (if not an obligation) to ask whether it is receiving anything for its investment other than good public relations for having an ethics committee. If committees are to argue that they, not clinical ethicists, are the best way to create a community of conscience (instead of being a conscience for the community), they must have evidence to support that claim. If they are to become an integral part of the institution, they must exist for reasons other than the members' personal growth and development. (Even though that is no small achievement, it nevertheless does not make the ethics committee an integral part of the institution; rather, the committee becomes an activity or a hobby club.)

The meaning and methods of evaluation need to be understood more broadly by committees. Evaluation need not be perceived as a way to judge (and punish) committees and committee members. At its best, evaluation can be a way to help committee members determine whether they are becoming more competent in this type of work and whether the committee as a whole is functioning in a way that makes a difference in the ethical climate of the hospital.

If committees want to help create a community of conscience to improve respect for human dignity in their institution (including the dignity of patients, families, staff, and physicians) on a day-to-day basis, they need to determine the best way to accomplish this. Only when ethics committees can see evaluation as something they can do *for* themselves and not *to* themselves, something that offers them an opportunity to do what they want to do better and more effectively, and something that can be quite interesting will they begin to respond positively to internal or external calls for such an exercise.

This chapter focuses on the self-evaluation of ethics committees and their work. Discussion centers on evaluation as a tool for thinking about how the committee can work better for both its members and its constituency. The process should involve surveying ethics committee members and clients to solicit their perceptions.

Summative and Formative Evaluation

Evaluation is often described as summative or formative evaluation. *Summative evaluation* focuses on the product, that is, how well the ethics committee is doing its job. If the hospital is investing dollars in the ethics committee, is it getting its money's worth? How good is the committee at doing what it says it is doing (and presumably what the institution has charged it to do)? Has the presence of the committee in the hospital led to fewer ethical problems? To increased staff understanding of ethical guidelines and consensus? To more satisfied patients? To fewer lawsuits? To less frustrated nursing staff? To lower staff turnover? A summative evaluation, then, serves to determine how successfully the committee has achieved the goals it set out to achieve.

Formative evaluation, on the other hand, looks at the process, that is, whether the ethics committee is conducting its activities in the appropriate manner (whatever that manner may be). This form of evaluation is less concerned with whether the committee is achieving its goals than with whether the processes created by, or imposed on, the committee are being followed and whether they can be improved. Committees operate on the assumption that their processes are appropriate for reaching the goals that would be measured by a summative evaluation. If that assumption is correct, to reach its goals the ethics committee must pay particular attention to how well those processes are functioning. Formative evaluation can also be seen as a kind of self-assessment in which the committee reflects on its activities and processes to determine how they can be improved.

Doing summative evaluation of ethics committees at this stage is likely to be unproductive. Given their many amorphous characteristics and the complex environment in which committees operate, it is virtually impossible to determine in any meaningful way whether they are doing a good job or to demonstrate that they make a difference in the hospital. However, it is possible to do formative evaluation to identify the committee's processes and to see whether those processes are followed and improved.

Identification of Goals and the Processes That Achieve Them

Despite a technical distinction between summative (goal-oriented) and formative (process-oriented) evaluation, evaluation/assessment in practice is similar to a set of Chinese boxes, in which one form of evaluation is enclosed in the other as the committee looks at processes and their various subprocesses and at goals and their various subgoals. Speaking primarily about the consultation function, Bernard Lo[1] argues that ethics committees should undergo strict evaluation before they are introduced as a standard "procedure" in hospitals. He proposes a series of goals for committees (in the form of the following questions) that include both formative and summative evaluation:

1. Are patients and their surrogates able to obtain review from committees?
2. Are committee recommendations given to those requesting assistance?
3. Are consultation recommendations consistent with the ethical consensus that currently exists in bioethics?
4. Are the disagreeing or inquiring parties satisfied with the ethics committees' involvement in these cases?

These are both formative and summative in the following sense. For example, the underlying assumption of the first question is that hospitals would be better places if patients were able to obtain assistance from ethics committees in dealing with their care when an ethical conflict or query arises. An ethics committee is then created whose goal is *either* to devise a process by which patients and their surrogates can obtain its assistance *or* to ensure that patients and their surrogates actually do request assistance from the ethics committee when they are experiencing a problem involving ethical aspects of their care.

To conduct a summative evaluation, the committee must know which of these goals is intended. If it is the first goal, evaluation would focus on whether the committee had created such a process; if it is the second, evaluation would focus on whether any patients or surrogates had in fact contacted the committee. If a formative evaluation were conducted, it would still be important to know which goal was intended. The committee would then look at the process that was intended to serve that goal. If the goal were to devise a process in which individuals could obtain access to the committee, it would look at how the process had been devised. For example, did the ethics committee obtain input from individuals in different disciplines? Did it consider patients' perceptions of the process? However, if the goal is to ensure that patients and their surrogates contact the committee, the committee would consider whether the process it devised is likely to be effective in making that possible.

It is reasonable to want to know both these things. Those who write about the need for ethics committee evaluation usually focus on summative evaluation. Do ethics committees work? Do they improve the situation in specific contexts? Sometimes, however, a summative evaluation is easy but not very helpful, whereas a formative evaluation would be wonderful to have but impossible to achieve.

For example, the goals of most committees are articulated either in a specific, rather simplistic manner (provide education, case review, and policy recommendations) or a somewhat vague and grand manner (improve the ethical climate of the institution or ensure proper respect for the dignity of patients and providers). In the first case, it is simple enough to determine whether the committee actually provided any education (regardless of how effective it was), case consultation (regardless of how thoughtful or effective it was), and policy recommendations (regardless of how knowledgeable or useful such recommendations were). For example, this is the kind of evaluation reported by Scheirton, in which she tracked the number of activities conducted by several ethics committees and correlated that number with the status ranking of the committee chairperson.[2] Although this kind of study is easy to do, the information it collects does not help us to know whether ethics committees either are a good idea or provide any benefit to anyone.

Specific goals are easy to evaluate, but the results of the evaluation are not very helpful. On the other hand, the vaguer, more grandiose committee goal statements are *not* easy (and perhaps even impossible) to evaluate, but if they could be, the evaluation would provide important information about ethics committees. Thus, if committees are going to attempt any evaluation, they must develop the kind of goals that both are easy to evaluate and allow for an evaluation that provides the committee with useful information. For example, suppose a committee develops a do-not-resuscitate (DNR) policy and a DNR form. It would be time-consuming and practically difficult to evaluate staff and physician knowledge of the new policy, but it would be relatively easy to determine correct use of the form. If the form is not used, or if it is used incorrectly, education can be targeted.

Goals can (and usually should) exist and be evaluated at every level of a specific activity. Unfortunately, committees are often content with an approach to evaluation that says: "They wanted us to recommend policies and we recommended three last year, so we are doing a good job." Such an approach may have been adequate at the beginning, but it will not be sufficient in the coming years if ethics committees are to (1) carry any weight in the institutional setting, (2) be entitled to a claim on institutional resources during a period of financial retrenchment, and (3) continue to hold their members' attention and interest.

Committee Self-Assessment

Committees can begin their evaluation with subjective self-assessment. Following are some questions that an ethics committee might use to evaluate itself on educating its members:

1. Has the ethics committee provided education to its members?
2. Did committee members learn what they should have learned (or learn anything particular) from the education provided by the committee?
3. What do members think they know relative to what they, as ethics committee members, should know?
4. What do they actually know relative to what they, as ethics committee members, should know?
5. Has self-education had any effect on the committee's work?

Has the Ethics Committee Provided Education to Its Members?

This question is easy to answer. The committee either has or has not had any intentionally designed self-education activity. Such activities might range from distributing articles to be discussed at meetings, to obtaining subscriptions to ethics journals for each member, to conducting formal didactic lectures during the meetings or at other times, to producing or attending educational conferences. Asking the question tells us something: if self-education is part of the committee's charge, we know whether the committee takes its charge seriously.

We might want to know something more. For example, how frequently do self-education activities take place? How much time is allotted? What form does the education take (lectures, articles, focused discussions)? How many members participate? These questions would more fully address this first question insofar as it refines quantitatively (as opposed to qualitatively) whether the committee provides education for its members. Sometimes these questions can verge on the normative if, for example, the question on form implies that some forms are better than others or if the question on time implies that a specified period of time is adequate for self-education. But suppose all these questions have been asked of the committee or at least of some responsible members. To the extent that these are factual questions, it is not necessary to obtain the entire committee's input. What should be done with this information as evaluation?

Herein lies the problem of ethics committee evaluation. The committee can look at this information and say, "Yes, we do self-education" or "No, we don't do self-education." But what then? Even committees that are not eager to pursue evaluation are likely to say: "Isn't whether we *do* self-education less important (because every committee does it) than whether the self-education we do *makes a difference?*" The committee could proceed to the second question.

Did Members Learn What They Should Have Learned from the Education Provided by the Committee?

This would require that the committee ask its members to relate what they had learned as a result of a particular self-education activity. Suppose the committee distributed an article on judgments about futile treatment for discussion at the meeting. At the end of the meeting (or at the end of the discussion), the committee members could be asked to fill in a brief form asking, for example, three things they had learned. The committee would then have evaluated the self-education activity with respect to what the members themselves judged they had learned. We must then again ask the question: what is to be done with this information?

It is not enough for the committee simply to ask the question, read through the responses briefly, and congratulate itself that its members report having learned something. Surely there is an implicit assumption that there are some things that are appropriate for the committee to learn in a specific activity. In choosing to distribute the article on judgments about medical futility, was the committee simply filling up committee time (too frequently the case) or did it have some goal, however implicit and unstated? Perhaps the goal was solely to expose members to someone's thinking on an issue of current interest in bioethics. Perhaps the goal was to compare this author's thoughts on the subject with the views of another author whose work committee members had previously discussed. Or perhaps it was to provoke the committee to think about its own sense of this issue and the appropriate response in the event the committee receives a case in which futility is a factor. The reason this article (instead of some other article) was distributed is at least part of the goal of this activity. To evaluate the activity, the goal must be specifically articulated. If the purpose of distributing this article is to compare one writer's analysis to another's and in reporting what he or she had learned no member of the committee mentions the earlier author's views, it would be proper to conclude that the particular goal was not met, although some other goals may have been.

Yet activities such as committee education are often conducted without any sense of goal other than the assumption that learning of some sort will take place if committee education activities are conducted. The committee leadership is often not too concerned with the nature of that learning. If that is the committee's attitude, evaluation tends to remain at question 1: did we do the activity? Failure to decide and articulate what the committee should be learning from specific activities (not least because to do so seems imperialistic/paternalistic/judgmental) and to communicate it to the rest of the committee poorly serves the members and the committee's mission. And it makes evaluation a difficult if not pointless activity.

What Do Members Think They Know or Actually Know Relative to What They Should Know?

An even more significant problem with evaluation is highlighted by the third and fourth questions. Both these questions imply that there is some standard or agreed-on body of knowledge that ethics committee members should possess. Although chapter 5 addresses this to some extent, there is in fact no agreed-on body of knowledge. The field of bioethics, as well as its subfield of ethics committees, lacks any organizing body or national association, and there is no one to prescribe the appropriate kind or amount of knowledge members should have. Over time, organizations will doubtless propose such standards,[3] but at present there is no consensus.

Therefore, to evaluate whether ethics committee members think they know (or can demonstrate that they know) what they should know, someone will need to specify what that knowledge should be. The committee itself could develop such a standard. To do so would depend heavily on members with more experience. But, simply having a committee ask itself "What does every person on this committee need to know in order for us to get on with our work?" should produce a wealth of information to committee leaders, not to mention considerable direction for those organizing the committee's self-education. If the committee goes so far as to decide at a basic level what all its members should know, it should then go on to develop evaluation measures to determine whether members in fact know these topics or think they know them. If members do not know them, the committee can develop a systematic education program to teach what needs to be learned.

After a period of time, the previously designed evaluation form could reassess whether the members now know what they previously did not. If members demonstrate knowledge, the evaluation has enabled the committee to know whether its education program worked. If they do not know, the committee must reexamine how it can conduct education more effectively. The evaluation will not, of course, tell the committee whether it was right about what its members *should* know, nor about whether that knowledge made any difference.

Has Self-Education Had Any Effect on the Committee's Work?

This particular evaluation is difficult to carry out. In order to do so, it first would be necessary to specify what effects the committee thought appropriate. Perhaps the committee could speculate that if every member had some basic knowledge of bioethics appropriate to an ethics committee, recommendations in case consultations would be more likely to conform to the "ethical consensus" that Lo speaks of and which is represented primarily in the Reports of the President's Commission for the Study of Ethical Problems in Medicine and Biomedical and Behavioral Research and in the body of statutory and case law in which general agreement on certain approaches is seen.[4-6] However, committee self-education and the achievement of basic knowledge are not the only factors that affect the outcome of case consultations, and it will be extremely difficult in practice to determine what factors contribute to what outcomes. Evaluating committee self-education in this format probably is not a very productive use of a committee's time and energies. But it often is the kind of evaluation that is imagined by either outsiders recommending evaluation or committees whose members feel that despite hard work and good intentions they will not be able to demonstrate the value of their work in an activity that is so complex and so dependent on personal interactions.

Results of Self-Assessment Tools

What could committees demonstrate that would be meaningful with respect to self-education? Following is a discussion of three surveys and how their results were applied.

Recent Author Survey

In a recent attempt to address the third question, the authors asked approximately 200 ethics committee members how they judged their knowledge of 24 topics. They were asked to rate their knowledge of each topic on a scale of 1 to 5, with 1 indicating they would feel comfortable teaching other ethics committee members about the topic and 5 indicating they had never heard of it as an issue in bioethics. The results of that survey are shown in figure 8-1.

Figure 8-1.   Bioethics Self-Evaluation Questionnaire Summary

	1 (%)	2 (%)	3 (%)	4 (%)	5 (%)
1 = Yes, I am very familiar with this topic and would feel comfortable teaching others about it.					
2 = Yes, I am familiar with this topic, but don't think I could answer questions about it.					
3 = Yes, I know about this topic in a general way, but not any of the specific issues.					
4 = No, I don't know much about this topic.					
5 = I've never even heard of this topic.					
1. Counseling for couples/pregnant women with regard to genetic disorders.	11	25	44	17	1
2. Pregnancy and abortion counseling for women with HIV infection.	16	29	34	18	1
3. Treatment of seriously ill newborns.	16	25	36	18	2
4. Baby Doe laws and regulations.	12	24	26	31	5
5. Use of infants with anencephaly as organ donors.	16	28	32	19	3
6. Whole brain death and neocortical death: definitions of death.	23	38	21	11	6
7. Confidentiality of medical records.	47	34	8	5	4
8. Violations of confidentiality with potentially dangerous patients.	21	37	20	16	4
9. Informed consent and assent for patients who are minors.	26	32	28	9	2
10. Informed consent for HIV testing.	32	39	19	4	3
11. Informed consent for innovative treatment.	20	35	26	14	4
12. Forgoing treatment for competent patients who are terminally ill.	43	32	15	2	5
13. Forgoing treatment for competent patients who are not terminally ill.	36	29	20	7	5
14. Forgoing treatment for incompetent patients who are terminally ill.	39	32	19	5	3
15. Forgoing treatment for incompetent patients who are not terminally ill.	30	30	23	9	4
16. Appropriate surrogates for incompetent patients.	28	33	27	8	2
17. Advance directives.	43	24	14	8	9
18. Medical determinations of futile treatment.	23	35	20	16	2
19. Do-not-resuscitate orders.	50	33	9	2	4
20. Pain control when adequate drug levels risk shortening life.	32	33	24	7	1
21. Euthanasia (or physician assistance in dying).	26	35	29	7	1
22. Surrogacy, including gestational surrogacy.	6	29	35	22	5
23. Refusal of blood for religious reasons (by adults, teens, children).	24	39	25	7	3
24. Sterilization (elective; competent and incompetent patients).	17	31	35	13	1

One purpose of this evaluation (or, more accurately, this self-assessment) was to have members think seriously about their knowledge of the 24 topics. We believed that ethics committee members might be expected to be reasonably familiar with most of them. The results were then returned to the committee so that members might see how their ethics committee scored generally, as well as how their scores compared to all ethics committee members who had responded to the survey. In this case, there was no intent to delineate an exclusive universe of topics about which ethics committee members might be expected to know. Rather, this was a selection of topics from that universe. Individuals also were asked to determine how important each one thought that topic was to his or her ethics committee.

A second purpose of this self-assessment was to enable ethics committees to see what their members thought they knew and where they felt some weakness, so the committee could then provide additional education if the topic was one that the committee thought important to its work. (For example, ethics committees in Catholic hospitals might know less about sterilization, in part because they might think the topic is not very important for them to know about.)

The survey was not intended to determine what members actually know. They may or may not be accurate in their perceptions of what they know, but we judged that they probably are accurate in their perceptions of what they do not know. In some instances, it also served to encourage those who conduct education for committees. For example, one committee that had devoted considerable time to self-education on ethical issues in the making of futility judgments scored significantly higher than the average on that topic. As one individual acknowledged, somewhat ruefully, "It doesn't mean they actually know more, but at least it means they think they know more. And given the amount of time we spent on that issue, they *should* think they know more."

Previous Evaluation Studies of Ethics Committees

The only published ethics committee evaluation studies appear to be rather broad in scope and oriented more toward summative than formative evaluation. It may be useful to describe them and to contrast their approaches to other approaches.

Two evaluation studies have been conducted by Hern.[7] In 1989, he surveyed the staff of a Denver hospital to help the ethics committee find out how physicians regarded the committee. He also wanted to find out how much ethics education physicians in the institution had received in recent years, including during medical school. Judging the committee required that the physicians actually have some knowledge of, and experience with, the committee (which they generally did not). As a result, the study actually focused more on how the physicians thought an ethics committee *should* function, leaving the committee itself to determine whether it met the physicians' expectations and, if not, how it could do so. In some senses, Hern's Denver study is similar to a focus group conducted by a business: trying to attract its audience, it looks to see what its audience wants, what will make it feel comfortable. Although this is a legitimate goal of evaluation, ethics committees might want to think about how well this approach will serve them in the long run.

In this particular hospital, physicians wanted the committee to provide lots of education, but were ambivalent about its becoming involved in case consultation. Although in theory the physicians saw case consultation as a useful function, in practice they found it somewhat threatening. The study's recommendations were wide-ranging, including a redefinition of committee goals, the inclusion of significantly more physicians in its membership so that they might better understand the committee's function, the establishment of permanent subcommittees to conduct consultation and institutional education, and the hiring of a part-time ethics coordinator.

In Hern's second study (coauthored with a physician and a philosopher),[8] he moved to evaluate not only an ethics committee but also an ethics institute (the Vrolyk Institute, Northridge Hospital, in Northridge, California). The evaluation extended beyond physicians' perceptions to include those of nurses, administrators, social workers, chaplains, and hospital volunteers. In this study, respondents were considerably more familiar with the committee's and the institute's work, and they were surveyed not only about what they thought ethics committees should do, but also about how well this particular committee and institute were doing.

Respondents who had attended the institute's regularly scheduled ethics grand rounds were questioned particularly about whether their attendance at those sessions had helped them to better understand the ethical aspects of several specific topics. (They were not questioned about actual learning, only about their perception of having better understanding.) In addition, physician and nurse respondents who had brought a case to the committee were asked whether their expectations were met and whether they were helped by the experience. Recommendations issuing from this evaluation were not as fundamental as those from the earlier study, but included a regular publication for hospital staff, better access to the committee for consultation, more education programs, and participation in employee orientation. The evaluators concluded that the committee was well thought of and the recommendations essentially were intended to build on that regard.

There is no question that Hern's studies helped the respective committees consider what they could do to strengthen their relationship with their communities. But it is certainly possible that a committee that is already struggling (which appeared to be the case with the Denver hospital committee) would be overwhelmed with the results of such a study and, rather than reevaluate its goals, would decide to disband and pursue some other activity. In the second case (the California hospital), the committee and supporting institute were in a much stronger position to accept criticism. For example, when respondents were asked how their hospital's ethics committee compared to committees in other local hospitals, the response was overwhelmingly positive: "the best in the area!" The committee members must have been aware of this kind of support and approval, which made criticisms and recommendations easier to consider and accept.

One of the lessons that might be learned from these two evaluations is that committees should consider how much capacity—emotional and practical—they have to respond to the potential results of their survey. For example, the first committee might have been better able to respond to a narrower set of questions. Because the committee was aware that it had relatively little physician participation, before asking physicians for evaluation, it might have been better advised to try to strengthen its physician component or to attempt to find out why physicians were reluctant to participate.

Design of Evaluation Instruments

In designing any kind of evaluation instrument, the committee should be clear about both the goals of the activity being evaluated and the purpose of evaluating that activity (that is, what will be done once the evaluation is completed). A simple format is best. Before conducting any evaluation activity, the committee or a subcommittee should formally ask and answer the following questions:

1. What do we want to know?
2. Why do we want to know it?
3. What would we do if we had an answer to our question?
4. To whom should we talk to find out the answer, and can we get to them?
5. What do we need to ask them?

What Do We Want to Know?

Hundreds of questions could be asked, ranging from "Why do the members choose to be on this committee?" to "What difference does this committee make in this hospital?" All of them are interesting to someone. But the important question is, "What do the members as a group want to know?" Try to find something that makes sense for the whole committee, not just for one or two people. If everyone is to have some investment in the outcome, everyone must be invested in the original question. In an informal survey of approximately 100 ethics committee members, the authors asked the committee members what each one wanted to know about his or her committee. A wide range of answers was received (see figure 8-2).

Why Do We Want to Know It?

The answers to this question are many: "It would be interesting. We're just curious. I don't know; it just seems as if it would be a good thing to know. If we knew, we could work to improve our effect in that area." Which seems the best reason to pursue a question? If you do not have a clear purpose for getting answers to specific questions, wait until you do know why you want to know it. Curiosity is a wonderful quality, but in a world of limited time, priorities should be set.

What Would We Do If We Had an Answer to Our Question?

It is easy to think of a question; it is fairly easy to think of good reasons why you would want to know the answer to it. It is extremely easy to think of how pleased you are going to be when the results demonstrate what a good job the committee is doing. But what are you prepared to do if the results suggest that something has not worked very well, that more work or a different kind of work is needed? If a committee is not prepared to do the fix-up work that might be necessary when the question is answered, there's little point in bothering to ask it.

To Whom Should We Talk to Find out the Answer, and Can We Get to Them?

Some questions require answers from people who are difficult to reach. Think seriously about whether it is worth conducting an evaluation if the data you can obtain will still leave you uncertain about the answer. For example, suppose you set out to obtain information from patients knowing in advance that you will not be able to reach most of them. Someone says, "Well, it will still be worthwhile talking to the ones that we can reach." Ask yourself whether this is true.

What Do We Need to Ask Them?

The questionnaire or survey instrument should be designed carefully. What information do you really need? Is it easy for people to answer? There is a fine line between making the questions easy to answer (so people can return it or fill it in fully) and reducing the information you get to meaninglessness. Do not use a questionnaire until you have tried it out on a few people and had them tell you where they had problems with the questions. What is obvious to you will not be obvious to them.[9]

Evaluation/self-assessment requires a considerable investment of time and energy. Having invested that time and energy, however, nothing is more discouraging than to find out that the information is filed away (should anyone ever inquire whether the committee evaluates its activities) and little else is done with it. For example, the subcommittee of one ethics committee that conducted a one-month-before-and-one-year-after assessment of the effects of a new DNR policy (including a review of over 200 charts) found the whole committee generally uninterested in the results or in doing any kind of educational follow-up to determine how to make the policy work better. This kind of response did not further the committee's willingness to spend additional time on evaluation activities. It is also discouraging to think that a committee would be so little interested in trying to ensure that its work was effective.

Figure 8-2. What Would You Like to Know about Your Ethics Committee?

1. Documentation requirements for case review sessions.
2. Each member's personal beliefs and interests without having to follow administrative line.
3. How much we know about the major current ethical issues.
4. How well we do in case review.
5. What the image of our committee is in the hospital community.
6. If we are doing the most useful (important) things to prepare the members for effective participation.
7. What motivates a member to attend or not attend meetings.
8. Whether the staff and medical community see us as nonthreatening.
9. What the benefit of having an ethics committee is to the doctors on their practice, their relationship to hospital staff, and their relationship to their patients.
10. Whether each member of this committee has a clearly defined idea of the purpose of our committee.
11. Whether the members of this committee feel our purpose is being achieved.
12. Whether we are actually providing education to hospital staff or whether staff just "tolerate" the ethics input.
13. Whether the committee is perceived as a policing committee in the institution at large.
14. How physicians are selected for membership on the committee.
15. How we can discuss topics the cochairperson does not really want to handle.
16. Whether our committee should have a more structured orientation for new members.
17. Whether the agenda should be sent out ahead of time.
18. How the committee could let the rest of the hospital staff know what goes on in our meetings.
19. Whether members feel satisfied with the outcomes of the committee.
20. If the committee is headed in the right direction.
21. If members feel they have an equal right to speak.
22. How much authority the committee has to affect the institution.
23. What we want our committee to look like in five years.
24. How the chairperson was chosen.
25. Why we do not do case consultation.
26. How aware the members are of the goals and accomplishments of the committee.
27. What the major motivation is for continuing to serve on the committee.
28. More about the hidden agendas.
29. What members think about having regular, open forum committee meetings.
30. What members think about making the committee a communitywide structure.
31. Whether family and residents know of our existence and how to access us in case of need.
32. Whether the committee is a comfortable group to access if a health care provider has an ethical dilemma.
33. Whether health care providers want to know more about what is legally "correct" or ethically "correct" in a given situation.
34. Why physicians are not more comfortable with the consultation process.
35. How important the ethics committee is to the hospital.
36. What members expect of the committee.
37. What members do after they leave meetings.
38. Whether members know about the ethics committee's policy and procedures.
39. Whether members have agendas they want solved based on personal experience.
40. Why they joined the committee.
41. Whether everyone feels heard. What barriers are felt to expression of disagreement.
42. What depth of understanding they have about the issues discussed.
43. What they mean when they use terms like *beneficence* or *autonomy*.
44. Whether there is a strong interest in continuing to participate on the committee.
45. Whether we are staying focused on ethics issues or have gotten sidetracked.
46. Whether we are benefiting from the knowledge and expertise of our members and really getting to know one another.
47. Whether this committee can be effective without involvement of physicians through attendance and participation.
48. Whether members look forward to monthly meetings.
49. Whether members feel being on the committee is worth their time.
50. Whether members think our chairperson is competent.
51. Why attendance is dwindling at meetings.
52. Why more people in the hospital do not know about the committee.
53. What members want to learn.
54. Whether everyone on the committee sees a benefit to having the committee and really wants to be there.
55. Whether members respect each other.
56. Whether we can really promote change or make a difference.
57. How committed the hospital president is to this committee.
58. What our priorities are.

Figure 8-2. (Continued)

59. How much time we are willing to commit to our goals.
60. Why members are chosen the way they are.
61. How the committee interacts with other hospital committees.
62. Whether we are addressing anybody's needs.
63. Whether we get input from all facets of the hospital.
64. Whether committee members should be required to have specific professional backgrounds.
65. Whether members should volunteer or be appointed.
66. What the medical staff/administration wants regarding committee development.
67. Who educates the committee members.
68. Whether our committee is unbiased.
69. How much self-study the committee members do, and in what areas.
70. What cases should be reviewed by the committee.
71. How to deal with money issues in cases.
72. How we can educate our members to look at ethical issues, not just legal ones.
73. Whether we are keeping up with issues in the field.
74. Whether members know when they have made a contribution.
75. Whether families who have interacted with the committee benefited.
76. Why we do not have minority representation. Whether others on the committee feel that is a deficit.
77. Whether members say what they really think or what they think everybody else wants to hear.
78. How to know when consensus is reached.
79. What the quiet people think about the committee.
80. Why I was asked to be on the committee.
81. How the chairperson could be more effective.
82. Whether people are more concerned with product or process.
83. Whether enough consideration is given to process versus good or bad product.
84. Whether too much authority is given to the opinions of physicians.

Categories for Evaluation Tasks

If a careful delineation of goals is the critical factor in conducting any kind of self-assessment or evaluation, what kinds of goals should ethics committees be considering as part of some modest evaluation project? The authors propose that evaluation should be divided into a number of discrete categories: education, consultation, policy writing, membership selection, committee leadership, and committee process. Following are some goals (provided as questions to be answered) that might be specified for each of these categories:

Education

1. What do members think is the basic body of information they should possess?
2. Are members familiar with a basic body of information?
3. Do members judge themselves to be familiar with a basic body of information?
4. Do individual educational activities have specific learning goals?
5. Does the committee have a well-developed and systematic educational plan for either itself or the hospital community that includes learning objectives for both each activity and the overall plan?
6. Is the committee's educational plan carried out in a systematic way?
7. Does the committee know the educational needs of the hospital community?
8. Do the recipients of committee education learn the relevant information from educational programs?

Consultation

1. Does the committee have a well-considered consultation protocol?
2. Does the committee follow its consultation protocol?
3. Do hospital staff and physicians know that the committee does case review?

4. Do staff and physicians think the committee does competent case review?
5. What is the sense of those who have brought cases to the committee with regard to their experience?
6. Are case consultation recommendations consistent with the bioethics consensus referred to by Lo?[10]
7. How would other ethics committees respond to the same case if it were brought to them?
8. What do the members of this ethics committee think about how the committee has handled specific case reviews?
9. Do patients/families know about the availability of case review?
10. Do patients/families think that case review would ever be of help to them?

Policy Writing

1. Do hospital staff and physicians know about the policies the committee has written?
2. Do staff and physicians understand the policies (or a specific policy) the committee has written?
3. Do staff and physicians agree with the appropriateness of the content and procedure in hospital policies?
4. Is the policy followed?
5. Are patients/families concerned about hospital policies?
6. How do the policies written by this committee compare to those written by other hospital ethics committees on the same topic?
7. What policies do staff and physicians think are needed in this hospital?
8. Do we follow our process for writing policies? (What would such a process be?)
9. Are our policies consistent in terms of form? (What form should they have?)

Membership Selection

1. Is our committee genuinely multidisciplinary?
2. Does our committee function in terms of its multidisciplinarity?
3. What functions are the different disciplines to serve on this committee?
4. Do our members know why they were chosen?
5. What is the best way to obtain members from many disciplines?
6. Do our members have the skills and attitudes we need?
7. How do we select new members for the committee?
8. How should we remove from the committee those who are not interested? Not contributing? Retarding our progress?

Committee Leadership

1. Do members support the committee leadership?
2. Do committee members agree about who are committee leaders?
3. Does the committee support the process by which leaders are selected?
4. By what process should leaders be selected?

Committee Process

1. Do members enjoy our meetings?
2. Do we achieve something at meetings? (Do our meetings have a sense of purpose?)
3. What should we be accomplishing at meetings?
4. What would a trained outside observer think of our meetings?
5. Does our committee agree about the kind of group process that is important for this committee?
6. Does our committee agree about the importance of group process for this committee?

7. Does our group process reflect our commitment to multidisciplinary process?
8. How would an independent outside observer describe our group process?
9. Does our committee function as a group of equals?
10. Does our committee demonstrate its concern for members as individuals?
11. Does our committee's group process affect attendance, membership retention, or member satisfaction? Interest of potential new members?

A series of assessment tools is included in figures 8-3 through 8-8 (pp. 126–31). These can be used directly or combinations of questions can be selected to be used in a specifically designed assessment tool for the individual committee. Some questions might be posed two ways: *should* we do X? and *do* we do X? It is possible that, even on questions that seem relatively factual (for example, does (should) everyone participate in meeting discussions?), there will be disagreement about both the factual question and the normative question. Before embarking on an assessment exercise, however, the committee should discuss its reason for doing it, the specific goal of the evaluation, and what is to be done with the information provided by the evaluation. A useful adage for evaluation is "Don't ask questions if you don't want to hear the answers or if you don't want to respond to the answers."

Conclusion

A number of writers have strongly argued that ethics committees need to become accountable for their work and that evaluation of committees should be forthcoming. It is both puzzling and frustrating to hear this at a time when even reliable data about the number of ethics committees in the United States or about their location do not exist. Significant external evaluation will surely have to await the collection of basic objective data. However, committees can and should develop the habit of at least informally evaluating their own work, clarifying and articulating the goals of their various activities, and specifying what processes will lead them to those goals.

Because evaluation for ethics committees is a new phenomenon, everyone still has much to learn about it. We would urge committees that do embark on evaluation activities to share their experiences with other committees through ethics committee networks, ethics committee newsletters and journals, and electronic bulletin boards (such as those operated by the Center for Healthcare Ethics, St. Joseph Health System, in Orange, California, and the Michigan Educational Resource Network, Michigan State University, in East Lansing, Michigan). Both methods of evaluation and the results of evaluation need to be communicated so that committees can learn what kind of evaluation is most helpful.

Figure 8-3. Meetings Assessment

Please circle the appropriate number indicating your response to each of the following statements. The numerical responses represent a continuum in which 1 = agree strongly and 5 = disagree strongly.

	Agree				Disagree
1. I look forward to going to ethics committee meetings.	1	2	3	4	5
2. It's important that meetings begin on time.	1	2	3	4	5
3. I attend most meetings.	1	2	3	4	5
4. Every meeting should have an agenda.	1	2	3	4	5
5. I like receiving the agenda before the meeting.	1	2	3	4	5
6. Our meetings follow the agenda.	1	2	3	4	5
7. I usually read the minutes before the meeting.	1	2	3	4	5
8. I know how the meeting agenda is planned.	1	2	3	4	5
9. I have occasionally asked to have an item placed on the agenda.	1	2	3	4	5
10. Meetings should end at the scheduled time.	1	2	3	4	5
11. Our meeting room is conducive to group work.	1	2	3	4	5
12. Every meeting should include an education section.	1	2	3	4	5
13. Discussions at our meetings tend to be dominated by one group (for example, doctors, nurses, chaplains, administrators, ethicists).	1	2	3	4	5
14. Our committee makes too many decisions by voting.	1	2	3	4	5
15. Our committee makes too many decisions by consensus.	1	2	3	4	5
16. Case recommendations should always be voted on.	1	2	3	4	5
17. Administrative decisions should always be voted on.	1	2	3	4	5
18. Our committee has representatives from as many professional disciplines as we need.	1	2	3	4	5
19. Our committee's actions reflect a multidisciplinary view.	1	2	3	4	5
20. Our committee would benefit from meeting more often.	1	2	3	4	5
21. This committee would do as well if it met less often.	1	2	3	4	5
22. Our meetings are too short.	1	2	3	4	5
23. Our meetings are too long.	1	2	3	4	5
24. Our meetings are about the right length of time.	1	2	3	4	5
25. I leave most meetings feeling that we have achieved something.	1	2	3	4	5
26. We should fill out a brief evaluation form at the end of each meeting.	1	2	3	4	5
27. This committee is more interesting than other hospital committees to which I belong.	1	2	3	4	5
28. Our meetings are planned very well.	1	2	3	4	5
29. This committee effectively establishes meeting priorities.	1	2	3	4	5

Comments:

Figure 8-4. Group Process Assessment

Please circle the appropriate number indicating your response to each of the following statements. The numerical responses represent a continuum in which 1 = agree strongly and 5= disagree strongly.

	Agree ——————— Disagree
1. New committee members or guests are always introduced.	1 2 3 4 5
2. Members are always introduced to guests or new members.	1 2 3 4 5
3. Introductions aren't limited just to name and profession or work location.	1 2 3 4 5
4. Every member usually speaks during a meeting.	1 2 3 4 5
5. I feel easy about entering into committee discussions.	1 2 3 4 5
6. Our committee's atmosphere makes it easy to participate.	1 2 3 4 5
7. No member(s) dominate the discussions at meetings.	1 2 3 4 5
8. Our committee is frustrating because some members are so domineering.	1 2 3 4 5
9. I feel I know most people on the committee better than I did when I first joined the committee.	1 2 3 4 5
10. Some members are more central to the committee's functioning than others.	1 2 3 4 5
11. Every committee needs a core group to run it.	1 2 3 4 5
12. I am important to the functioning of this committee.	1 2 3 4 5
13. I feel comfortable calling other members by their first names.	1 2 3 4 5
14. I believe all members should be addressed by title.	1 2 3 4 5
15. I think group exercises (role-play, consciousness-raising sessions, personal value discussions, group evaluation) make committees better.	1 2 3 4 5
16. Our committee would benefit from an all-day retreat.	1 2 3 4 5
17. I have made new friends on this committee.	1 2 3 4 5
19. I feel at home on this committee.	1 2 3 4 5
20. I think I know how most people on this committee will respond to a controversial situation (for example, legalization of active euthanasia, gestational surrogacy).	1 2 3 4 5
21. I would like to belong to this committee for a long time.	1 2 3 4 5
22. I have suggested to colleagues that they join the committee.	1 2 3 4 5
23. I believe that our members say what they honestly think and feel when a difficult situation or case arises.	1 2 3 4 5
24. After a difficult situation/case is discussed, small groups of members tend to stay around to continue discussing it.	1 2 3 4 5
25. This ethics committee is a more cohesive group than when I first joined it.	1 2 3 4 5
26. This committee is very effective in this institution.	1 2 3 4 5
27. This committee is well known in this facility.	1 2 3 4 5

Comments:

Figure 8-5. Leadership Effectiveness Assessment

Please circle the appropriate number indicating your response to each of the following statements. The numerical responses represent a continuum in which 1 = agree strongly and 5 = disagree strongly.

	Agree —————— Disagree
1. This committee has effective leadership.	1 2 3 4 5
2. A committee's leadership should change regularly.	1 2 3 4 5
3. Having cochairpersons helps a committee run better.	1 2 3 4 5
4. Restricting committee leadership to physicians makes the committee less effective.	1 2 3 4 5
5. Electing leaders is the best way to decide leadership.	1 2 3 4 5
6. On this committee the elected/appointed officers are not the only committee leaders.	1 2 3 4 5
7. Committee chairpersons should be experts in bioethics.	1 2 3 4 5
8. It takes special skills to be a committee chairperson.	1 2 3 4 5
9. Every person on the committee should have an equal chance to become a committee leader.	1 2 3 4 5
10. Our committee supports education for people who want to become part of the committee's leadership.	1 2 3 4 5
11. I know who the leaders in this committee are.	1 2 3 4 5
12. I would like to become a leader in this committee.	1 2 3 4 5
13. Our leaders establish specific committee goals each year.	1 2 3 4 5
14. Our leaders help us keep in touch with the broader field of bioethics.	1 2 3 4 5
15. Our committee chairperson(s) conducts meetings very effectively.	1 2 3 4 5
16. Committees should have subcommittees so that more people have an opportunity to take on responsibility.	1 2 3 4 5
17. We have selection criteria for our leaders.	1 2 3 4 5
18. Our criteria for leaders are drawn from our own standards, not from the hospital culture.	1 2 3 4 5
19. A committee with good leaders should stick with them.	1 2 3 4 5

Comments:

Figure 8-6. Membership Issues Assessment

Please circle the appropriate number indicating your response to each of the following statements. The numerical responses represent a continuum in which 1 = agree strongly and 5 = disagree strongly.

	Agree ——————— Disagree
1. When selecting ethics committee members, we should look for individuals with special skills.	1 2 3 4 5
2. When selecting committee members, we should look for individuals with special attitudes.	1 2 3 4 5
3. Ethics committee members should master a body of knowledge before joining the committee.	1 2 3 4 5
4. Committee members should master a body of knowledge within a year of joining the committee.	1 2 3 4 5
5. I know how members are selected for my committee.	1 2 3 4 5
6. Ethics committee members should be rotated off the committee after a specified period of time.	1 2 3 4 5
7. Members should stay on the committee as long as they want, if they attend and participate appropriately.	1 2 3 4 5
8. Some individuals should be permanent members and others should rotate off the committee after a specified period of time.	1 2 3 4 5
9. The ethics committee should provide all necessary education for its members.	1 2 3 4 5
10. All ethics committee members should attend ethics conferences at least occasionally.	1 2 3 4 5
11. I can identify committee members who are particularly skillful at case review/consultation.	1 2 3 4 5
12. I can identify committee members who are particularly skillful at writing policies and guidelines.	1 2 3 4 5
13. I can identify committee members who are particularly skillful at providing education.	1 2 3 4 5
14. Committee members should receive some kind of credit for being on the committee.	1 2 3 4 5
13. Some people at this institution can't be on the committee because they can't get time off to attend.	1 2 3 4 5
14. Most members of this committee take the committee's work seriously.	1 2 3 4 5
15. We have the right people on our ethics committee.	1 2 3 4 5
16. The ethics committee should have a significant number of members who have power in the institution.	1 2 3 4 5
17. I am satisfied with the members' skills and knowledge.	1 2 3 4 5
18. Our committee has good representation from many different disciplines.	1 2 3 4 5

Comments:

129

Figure 8-7. Prospective Case Review Assessment

Please circle the appropriate number indicating your response to each of the following statements. The numerical responses represent a continuum in which 1 = agree strongly and 5 = disagree strongly.

	Agree———Disagree				
1. Case review should be done by the entire committee.	1	2	3	4	5
2. Case review should be done by a small group chosen for their skills.	1	2	3	4	5
3. Case review should be done by a small group drawn from all members of the committee.	1	2	3	4	5
4. Case review should be done by a single skilled person.	1	2	3	4	5
5. The committee should have a written procedure that guides the members in doing case review.	1	2	3	4	5
6. The committee should keep written records of cases it reviews.	1	2	3	4	5
7. The committee should always write a chart note.	1	2	3	4	5
8. The committee should write a chart note if the attending physician requests it to do so.	1	2	3	4	5
9. The committee should inform other hospital committees (for example quality assessment, risk management, chief of staff, chief executive officer) of the outcome of some cases.	1	2	3	4	5
10. Making recommendations in case review intimidates the physicians and others involved in the patient's care.	1	2	3	4	5
11. Offering a forum for discussing a case doesn't really help anyone get matters resolved.	1	2	3	4	5
12. People who ask the committee to become involved in a case should have to give informed consent to the procedure.	1	2	3	4	5
13. Case reviews should not be done without the attending physician being present.	1	2	3	4	5
14. Case reviews should not be done without the patient's or surrogate's consent.	1	2	3	4	5
15. Case reviews should always be formally and systematically evaluated.	1	2	3	4	5
16. Subcommittees that do case review should always report what they have done to the whole committee.	1	2	3	4	5
17. I understand our committee's *purpose* for doing case review.	1	2	3	4	5
18. I am confident in our committee's case review *process.*	1	2	3	4	5
19. Case review is the most important function of ethics committees.	1	2	3	4	5
20. The committee activity I am most interested in is case review.	1	2	3	4	5
21. I usually feel good about the case review done by our committee.	1	2	3	4	5
22. Many ethical problems in patient care at our hospital are never addressed.	1	2	3	4	5
23. In our hospital, people know that we offer case review.	1	2	3	4	5
24. Those who have come to the committee have been quite satisfied with the committee's ability to help them.	1	2	3	4	5
25. I wish our committee did more case review.	1	2	3	4	5
26. Our committee needs more education on how to do good case review.	1	2	3	4	5
28. Our committee would benefit from training in mediation or other conflict resolution skills.	1	2	3	4	5
29. I am concerned about liability in doing case review.	1	2	3	4	5
30. I am usually satisfied with my part in case review.	1	2	3	4	5
31. I think clinicians at the bedside can do a better job of resolving ethical issues than ethics committees.	1	2	3	4	5

Comments:

Figure 8-8. Policy and Guidelines Assessment

Please circle the appropriate number indicating your response to each of the following statements. The numerical responses represent a continuum in which 1 = agree strongly and 5 = disagree strongly.

	Agree———————Disagree				
1. Our committee has written all the policies this institution needs.	1	2	3	4	5
2. Our committee spends too much time writing policy.	1	2	3	4	5
3. Policy writing is the most important function of the ethics committee.	1	2	3	4	5
4. The best way to handle policies would be if some other group in the institution wrote them and then sent them to the ethics committee for review.	1	2	3	4	5
5. The best way to handle policies would be for a small group of ethics committee members to work on them and bring them to the whole committee only when they were ready to be approved.	1	2	3	4	5
6. Policies in our institution should all have the same format.	1	2	3	4	5
7. Our committee doesn't provide enough education on new or revised policies.	1	2	3	4	5
8. If we write a new policy or revise an old one, we should provide education on the policy throughout the hospital.	1	2	3	4	5
9. If we write a new policy or revise an old one, we should organize some way of finding out whether the new/revised policy is understood by the staff/physicians.	1	2	3	4	5
10. If we write a new policy or revise an old one, we should organize some way of finding out whether the policy is being followed.	1	2	3	4	5
11. The ethics committee is the best group to determine what policies are needed or need to be revised.	1	2	3	4	5
12. The staff/physicians are the best people to determine what policies are needed or need to be revised.	1	2	3	4	5
13. No one knows the policies anyway, so it's a waste of time to write them or revise them.	1	2	3	4	5
14. Policies are written to protect the hospital legally.	1	2	3	4	5
15. If we found out that a policy wasn't working, our ethics committee would do something about it.	1	2	3	4	5
16. Policy evaluation is a good use of the committee's time.	1	2	3	4	5
17. Policies should never be discussed by the whole committee because members only argue about wording.	1	2	3	4	5
18. Our committee does a good job of writing and revising policies.	1	2	3	4	5
19. Our committee does a good job of providing education on new and revised policies.	1	2	3	4	5
20. Our committee does a good job of evaluating new and revised policies.	1	2	3	4	5

Comments:

Notes and References

1. Lo, B. Behind closed doors: promises and pitfalls of ethics committees. *New England Journal of Medicine* 317(1):46–50, 1987.

2. Scheirton, L. Determinants of hospital ethics committee success. *HEC Forum* 4(6):342–59, 1992.

3. See, for example, Callahan, D., and Thornton, B. *Bioethics education: expanding the circle of participants.* Briarcliff Manor, NY: The Hastings Center, 1992.

4. President's Commission for the Study of Ethical Problems in Medicine, Biomedical and Behavioral Research. *Defining Death.* Washington, DC: United States Government Printing Office, 1981.

5. President's Commission for the Study of Ethical Problems in Medicine, Biomedical and Behavioral Research. *Deciding to Forego Life-Sustaining Treatment.* Washington, DC: U.S. Government Printing Office, 1983.

6. Society for the Right to Die. *Right to Die Court Decisions.* Vols. 1–3. New York City: Society for the Right to Die, 1993.

7. Hern, H. G., Jr. A study of physician attitudes and perceptions of a hospital ethics committee: and ethics and human values committee survey. *HEC Forum* 2(2):105–25, 1990.

8. Hern, H. G., Jr., Rain, L., and Vrolyk, A. Hospital staff perceptions of the ethics committee and the bioethics institute: a multidisciplinary approach. *HEC Forum* 3(3):129–46, 1991.

9. Sudman, S., and Bradburn, N. M. *Asking Questions: A Practical Guide to Questionnaire Design.* San Francisco: Jossey-Bass, 1983.

10. Lo.

9

The Law: Lawyers as Members and Member Liability

One of the hallmarks of contemporary medical practice in the United States is its preoccupation with the law—particularly with regard to malpractice suits. It is not surprising, then, that hospital ethics committees also share the concerns implicit in that preoccupation. One of the first questions asked at every ethics committee conference is: "Should we have a lawyer on the committee?" However, it is not clear whether the real sense of that question is: "Do we have to have a lawyer?" or "May we have a lawyer?" or "Do we need a lawyer?" Ethics committees appear to be both attracted to and repelled by lawyers (for example, the same question is rarely asked about nurses, administrators, philosophers, clergy, or social workers) and their ambivalence as to how to relate to lawyers and the law is apparent in this too frequently asked question.[1]

This chapter discusses whether it is necessary for committees to include a lawyer as a member and what his or her role might be. It also provides some basic information on the potential liability of both the ethics committee as a whole and its individual members. Although this chapter does not provide a comprehensive analysis of liability issues, it should help members gain some idea of the possible problems, the probability of those problems arising, and the liability issues those problems pose. An attorney member, if the committee has one, can provide further education if the committee feels a need for it or can help to remind members of these issues.

A Lawyer on the Committee

Ethics committees should have some knowledge of the law, even though their primary business is that of analyzing ethical issues and not legal issues. The questions in the following subsections might be helpful to committees that are considering asking a lawyer to become a member.

Should the Lawyer Have the Appropriate Personal Qualities?

An attorney on the ethics committee could be helpful in clarifying legal issues and tracking legal developments if the other committee members do not feel confident about their abilities in this area—including their ability to know when to ask a lawyer for advice or assistance. However, the lawyer selected should have the same personal qualities required of other committee members: an openness to discussion, a willingness to participate, the ability to listen to others, the ability to focus on the goals and charge of the ethics committee, and an interest in the ethical aspects of health care. A lawyer who has those qualities would genuinely enrich the ethics committee's ability to do its work.

If the committee has a choice (and it does not in some institutions), it should have a lawyer on the committee only if those forming or belonging to the committee believe they can find an individual who possesses the personal qualities requisite for *any* good ethics committee member. If they cannot find such a lawyer, they would likely be better off without one as a member. In this event, during the course of its work, the committee would need to remember to obtain advice about the law should it impinge on what they are doing. Seeking the advice of outside legal counsel as needed is preferable, because many people have difficulty distinguishing between law and ethics and a lawyer on the committee who sees himself or herself as the sole or ultimate arbiter of what is legal is likely to have a chilling effect on the committee process and its thinking about ethics. Furthermore, there are committees without a lawyer as a regular member that seem to function quite well.

Should the Lawyer Be from within or outside the Institution?

Which of the many lawyers who would be helpful to the committee should be asked to join? That is, should the committee look to the institution's lawyer or to a lawyer practicing outside the particular hospital or even outside health care law entirely? It may not be appropriate to have the hospital's attorney as a regular member of the committee, because that person may be put in an uncomfortable position in terms of his or her responsibility to the overall facility. In other words, because the hospital's attorney has a professional responsibility to protect the interests of the institution rather than those of the patients (even though those interests often may be identical), his or her being a member of the ethics committee could result in a potential conflict of interest. If the committee can locate no other attorney it feels comfortable with and confident about, or if, for other reasons, the facility's attorney *must* be a member of the committee, his or her role on the committee should be carefully delineated. Perhaps the most appropriate way to get around the conflict-of-interest problem is to have the attorney participate as an advisory but not a voting member, or for the attorney not to participate in votes or discussions where he or she feels a primary responsibility to protect the institution.

Should the Lawyer Be a Health Care Lawyer?

If the hospital's attorney is not chosen, would a committee be better off with a lawyer who has some professional experience in health care law or one who is interested in bioethics but not particularly familiar with the law pertaining to it? We have seen committees that have gone both ways on this and one choice does not appear to be better than the other. The attorney without health care law experience is more likely to provide a community-oriented voice rather than a health care professional perspective, but a health care lawyer is more likely to understand the thrust and fine points of current law relating to bioethics as well as recent case decisions and legislation.

What Should the Committee Want from the Lawyer?

Having selected a lawyer, the ethics committee needs to articulate to that person what it wants from him or her. Perhaps it is easier to understand what is meant by asking a nurse to provide a nursing perspective than by asking an attorney to provide a legal perspective. By *nursing perspective* we mean the viewpoint of a health care professional whose primary obligation is that of advocate for the patient, frequently in the context of the patient's family relationships. Although lawyers are certainly interested in rights, it is not clear that this is what is sought from them. Robyn Meinhardt argues that lawyers have a particular gift for ethics committees: "clarity of reasoning and expression . . . from the lawyer's training and practice in rooting out ambiguity and multiple meanings in legal documents." She believes that "the lawyer member of a bioethics committee will be able to use these skills to help other committee members focus on the relevant issues in their discussions of ethical problems and to point out areas of inconsistency in positions taken."[2]

The committee may want the lawyer to offer only those kinds of skills in his or her role on the committee. It may also want the lawyer to provide ongoing education on the law generally as it applies to bioethics or to specific cases and their meaning as they arise. In addition, committee members may want the lawyer to help them understand their own legal risks, that is, to function as an advisor to the committee on the legal implications for the committee and its members.

The first two areas are commonly understood as the lawyer's role on the committee. The third has received virtually no discussion in the literature, and we do not view it as a proper use of the attorney member, because he or she has not been hired by the committee to provide professional services. However, if there is a real risk of committee liability, someone should at least be reflecting on the relationship between what the committee is doing and its risk of liability exposure.

Potential Liability Concerns for Ethics Committees

There is only one recorded instance of an ethics committee and its individual members being named as defendants in a lawsuit. Although the plaintiff in that case, Elizabeth Bouvia, never pursued her action against the ethics committee to final decision or judgment, the mere filing of the case sent shudders through the bioethics community. The relief she sought—removal of a nasogastric feeding tube inserted without her consent but with the alleged concurrence of the ethics committee—was granted in the landmark case of *Bouvia v. Superior Court*.[3] After the summons and complaint had been filed in the case, and while depositions were being taken, the physicians stated that they were "acting under the orders of the ethics committee" in placing the tube. Accordingly, Ms. Bouvia's attorneys amended the complaint to include the ethics committee as defendants. Once the appellate court ordered removal of the feeding tube, Ms. Bouvia dropped the suit against the committee and its individual members.[4]

Because there was no judicial pronouncement regarding the liability of ethics committee members in that case, it is impossible to predict how that court, or any other, would formulate or decide issues of criminal or civil liability regarding committee actions, decisions, or recommendations. It should be remembered that in our legal system any person can file suit against any other at any time for anything. Whether actual liability will be found by the court, with judgment rendered for damages, is another matter.

The absence of other suits against ethics committees or their members reflects one of several possibilities: (1) Ethics committees are doing their job well, thoughtfully, thoroughly, sensitively, conscientiously, and with careful attention to proper procedure; (2) the likelihood of the success of such a lawsuit has been deemed low and/or the potential judgment for damages not worth the effort; (3) the right set of circumstances (egregious conduct on the part of the ethics committee) has not yet occurred; (4) the "harmed or injured" patient died without heirs or family to pursue an action; or (5) the survivors either were not aware of all the facts and the grounds for litigation or chose not to litigate.

The absence of litigation should not lead committees to assume they are immune from legal concerns. If the ethics committee issues a mandatory directive or requires particular actions on the part of the physician, "those who direct these tortious acts of another share the legal responsibility—ethics committees with the clearest potential for legal responsibility are those that have been invested with the greatest formal authority."[5]

But even when there are no mandatory directives, committees may be heard as speaking with compelling authority. Although the consensus is that committees are only advisory, they may appear to operate from a position of moral authority, if not as the officially authorized "conscience of the institution." Because of this, their deliberations and recommendations may place a heavy burden on those who consult them to follow committee advice or to come up with very good reasons why those recommendations should not be followed. Under those circumstances, the burden on ethics committee members to exercise their responsibility diligently and conscientiously becomes even greater. However, rather than worry about liability, the committee would be better off concentrating on detail, adequate preparation, carefully-thought-out procedures, and good documentation, as well as on regularly obtaining review of its work, both from within and outside the committee.

The following subsections provide a brief discussion of the various types of liability of which committees should be aware.

Criminal Liability

A finding of criminal liability arising out of the deliberations of ethics committee members is extremely unlikely. A violation of criminal law requires (1) performance of an act that is specified as a crime in the criminal code and (2) having the intent to perform this act. This could arise if the ethics committee participated in or concurred with a physician's action (or the action of any other health care provider) intentionally and directly to cause the death of a patient, or if it failed to take action to prevent such a death when members knew that death might occur and were presumed to have authority or responsibility to intervene. (It might seem that ethics committees often do this, for example, in case reviews involving forgoing life-sustaining treatment. However, in such cases the intention is *not* to cause the patient's death but to honor the patient's wishes or those of his or her surrogates, or to act in the best interest of the patient, given the burdens and benefits of treatment possibilities. The conditions might be met if, in a case review, the physician told the committee that the patient had requested a lethal dose of medication and that he or she was inclined to give it, and the committee either agreed with the physician or did nothing to advise against the act.) Similarly, were an ethics committee found to have intentionally engaged in a conspiracy to cause the death of a patient, the possibility of criminal liability for the homicide might also exist. However, it should be repeated that such charges are very unlikely and that any prosecutor would have a significant burden of proof to overcome — the presumption of innocence until proven guilty and the legal requirement for proving a criminal case beyond a reasonable doubt.

One area with some realistic potential for criminal liability problems for ethics committees is child abuse and elder abuse. Some state statutes make criminal liability a possibility if health care personnel have knowledge of such abuse and fail to report it to the appropriate authorities. Ethics committees need to obtain specific guidance from local legal counsel on the responsibilities imposed by their particular state statutes if, in the course of case review, they become aware of such abuse situations.

Civil Liability — Tort Law

Legal actions raising issues of civil liability include tort, contract, and civil rights violations. Civil rights actions are brought to court by persons who believe they have been injured or wronged (in contrast to criminal charges, which are brought to court by the state in the person of the district attorney or prosecutor). Civil actions customarily seek damages to be paid directly to the aggrieved party (or the estate or family if he or she has died).

It is tort law with which ethics committees need to be most concerned, although recent federal laws such as the Americans with Disabilities Act (ADA) impose duties not to discriminate that can apply to hospitalized patients. For example, some have argued that permanently unconscious patients are disabled individuals and that failing to continue life-sustaining treatment for them would violate their civil rights under the ADA. Similarly, failure to provide treatment for seriously ill newborns might be construed as a violation of the child's civil rights (or, alternatively, as criminal child abuse, as under the Child Abuse amendments passed subsequent to the Baby Doe controversies).

Torts fall into two general categories: intentional (where the harm is intended) and negligent (where there is no intent of harm).

Intentional Torts

Intentional torts relevant to health care include battery, abandonment, false imprisonment, and breach of confidentiality. The plaintiff in an intentional tort action must establish that the act occurred and that the defendant intended harm.

Battery and False Imprisonment

This is an area in which ethics committees might run afoul of the law, especially with respect to case consultation or review. The law defines *battery* as the intentional touching or striking of another, without consent. A battery can occur even though the individual touched is not aware of it at the time it actually happens. There is no requirement of damages because battery is an intentional tort—the mere fact of touching without consent can be the basis of the suit. Hospitals routinely obtain a patient's signature on a consent form at the time of hospital admission and/or in anticipation of a surgical procedure as a defense against a charge of battery. Consent is an absolute defense against a charge of battery. If an ethics committee concurred with a physician's decision to operate or to perform some other invasive procedure without the patient's consent, that might give rise to a charge of battery or, in the ethics committee's case, abetting a battery. (Had Elizabeth Bouvia pursued her case against the ethics committee, her attorneys would most likely have claimed that the committee abetted the battery of Ms. Bouvia in its support of the physician's decision to insert a nasogastric tube for feeding purposes, without her consent.)

Similarly, an ethics committee might be alleged to have abetted a false imprisonment if it urged or encouraged using restraints when the medical facts did not warrant such action. Legislatures are beginning to look at the use of restraints, particularly in nursing homes. Ethics committees should seek advice of local counsel to find out if there are particular laws controlling use of restraints (both chemical and physical) in their state.

Abandonment

Abandonment is a particular area of tort law that courts have applied to health care professionals. Abandonment has been found in situations where the patient's illness or need for medical care continued, although the physician (or other health care provider) had terminated the relationship in an abrupt and unilateral manner, without either arranging for another to provide that ongoing care or giving the patient an opportunity to find another care provider. In cases where abandonment has been alleged, some courts have interpreted it as being the "most unforgivable sin" of medical malpractice. Given the right set of circumstances, where a committee might be alleged to have concurred with a physician's decision to forgo treatment without patient/surrogate involvement in the decision, and the patient was essentially left without medical or other care needs being met, an allegation of abandonment might well be raised. However, under usual circumstances it is doubtful that a prudent, conscientious, thoughtful ethics committee would participate in such a situation. The relationship between claims that futile treatment need not be offered or continued and legal insistence that patients not be abandoned is, however, one that ethics committees may need to study.

Breach of Privacy and Confidentiality

The final area of potential exposure for ethics committees in tort law would be that of breaching patient privacy rights, including the confidentiality of patient information.[6] Patients come into the health care system expecting that the information they give to health care professionals will be kept confidential. Health care team members are expected to maintain that confidentiality and release information only to those who need to know it in order to participate adequately in the patient's health care.

Release of information without consent. Release of such information to others without the patient's specific permission and consent (except for certain police and public health situations) is a legal violation for which money damages may be sought. As part of its investigation and deliberations, the ethics committee may become aware of information that it would not otherwise be privy to. Accordingly, the requirements for maintaining the patient's confidentiality, particularly in such troublesome areas as decisions regarding terminal care, may constitute a significant burden for ethics committees. This area should not be treated lightly, even though, to date, it has not been the source of litigation. If ethics committees cannot behave "ethically" in respecting and maintaining the patient's privacy and confidentiality, they set a poor standard and role model for others in the health care arena who are less committed to ethical issues.

Circulation of patient information. Despite the traditional commitment to confidentiality, patient information often receives wide circulation in health care facilities, independent of the caregivers' need to know.[7] Ethics committee members should have a very good grasp of what constitutes a breach of confidentiality. Patients' privacy is invaded and confidentiality breached by releasing information that identifies the patient or makes him or her readily identifiable. This occurs most commonly in the following ways:

- Information about the patient is discussed at a committee meeting at which "public members" are present, that is, members who are not part of the health care team. (It is not entirely clear whether this is a breach of confidentiality. Public members of the committee should have special education with respect to their obligations in this area, and patients and their families who participate in case review should be informed that the committee has public members.)
- Information about the patient is revealed in the committee's written minutes, which find their way into general circulation.
- Information about the patient is revealed when the committee conducts an educational program using the patient as the case exemplar.
- Information about the patient is revealed by committee members who are discussing the case in public arenas such as corridors, coffee shops, elevators, and so on.

Case review. Confidentiality becomes particularly problematic when the ethics committee reviews a case and the patient/surrogate has not been informed about the review or consented to it. In the normal course of health care delivery, intimate revelations that patients make are noted by the physician or other member of the health care team in the patient's medical record. Those statements are available to all staff members on the unit (and possibly throughout the facility) who have contact with either the patient or his or her medical record. It is assumed that these details will not be revealed because staff know the importance of confidentiality. The patient will never realize how many individuals know of the confidences he or she has entrusted to the physician.

Ethics committee consultation that the patient has no knowledge of might fall into this category of disclosure. This is especially true if no change in treatment plan follows the committee review. In addition, it might be argued that ethics committee members would not necessarily be expected to be included in that group of hospital personnel with a need to know. Claims that ethics committee review constitutes a breach of confidentiality may therefore be legitimate. Whether a judge or jury would affirm that claim is questionable.

Consultation. "Curbstone" consultations between physicians are common. Here, there is an informal seeking of advice and at least some specific information about a patient is given to the consulting physician. The patient is not readily identifiable and is not examined by the second physician; there are no fees; and the second physician has no responsibility. Breach of confidentiality in the true legal sense probably does not occur in such a situation, although more formal ethics committee consultations are similar. Perhaps the best advice for ethics committees is to suggest to clinicians that they inform the patient/surrogate of the decision to seek an ethics committee consultation and, when discussing the case, not to release the patient's name or circulate documents that identify the patient. Prior to each consultation, committees should remind members of the importance of preserving confidentiality and of not discussing the case outside the committee meeting.

Education. Confidentiality may be breached in the course of education because so much education is based on case studies. If the committee intends to use a particular case as a model for its educational efforts in the facility, it should obtain the consent of all (patient/surrogate and even health care professionals), or so generalize the facts as to make the individuals involved not readily identifiable. Facts such as sex, race, age, specific diagnoses, family situations, and so on, should be altered to protect the patient's privacy and confidentiality. Similarly, the committee's record of its deliberations regarding particular cases should be kept confidential, and the patient not readily identified or identifiable, unless the committee's records are kept in locked files and are not easily accessible to hospital staff at large. Where entries are made by the committee (or its designee) into the patient's medical record, these must receive the same assurance of confidentiality as do other entries in that record.

Negligence

In health care, negligence most commonly involves malpractice. In a case of negligence, four elements must be proved: (1) a duty and/or a standard of care on the part of the defendant toward the injured party (plaintiff); (2) a failure to exercise that duty (or a breach of the standard of care); (3) the existence of a proximate causal relationship between that failure or breach and the injury to the plaintiff; and (4) actual harm or injury, which can be measured in terms of money damages. In a medical malpractice action, the standard of care generally is held to be that level of care or performance that the well-trained, prudent physician (or similarly trained professional) would exercise under the same or similar circumstances. Expert witnesses are called to testify whether the conduct breached the standard.

Ethics committees also might be involved in negligence actions, based on a claim that a duty was owed by the committee to the patient, that the committee was required to conform to a standard of care in its deliberations, and that it deviated from that standard of care and thereby caused the patient damages. To establish the standard of care, expert witnesses would have to testify on the standard of care for ethics committees and whether the committee's actions deviated from it. In view of the fact that ethics committees have now existed for a considerable length of time across the country, diligent attorneys (for plaintiff and defense) would doubtless be able to find such experts to testify. However, it is unclear what that testimony would be. That ethics committees are not themselves treatment decision makers is, at least arguably, a standard for ethics committees. Beyond that, much is still in flux.

Liability for Interhospital Ethics Committee Activity

There are occasionally suggestions that one hospital's ethics committee serve as a consultant to another hospital or another hospital's ethics committee. The following comments on such practices should be considered. There is no apparent authority for the second hospital to cover (under its malpractice insurance) the visiting ethics committee members, because they are not employees of that hospital and would not normally be covered under a "vicarious liability" theory in which the employing hospital is responsible for the actions of its employees. Furthermore, there would be no authority for the first hospital to cover the actions of the "loaned" ethics committee members, because by operating in another hospital, they are outside the scope of their normal authority.

If this kind of interhospital consulting is to take place, the ethics committee of hospital A should obtain a letter either from its own facility's counsel stating that its activities will be covered or from the inviting facility's counsel stating that hospital B will cover the activities of the ethics committee when it is operating, by invitation, in that facility.

Peer Review Issues

Ethics committees are occasionally involved in cases in which physicians are violating patients' rights or wishes. In challenging the physician, the committee might expose itself to charges of defamation of character by the physician, particularly if the committee did anything of a whistle-blowing nature, such as reporting the physician up the chain of command. However, relevant state law might see the ethics committee as a peer review committee, which would mean that it was immune from prosecution, assuming it acted in good faith and without malice. Peer review statutes may provide some liability protection for ethics committee members if they meet the statutory definition of *a covered committee* (one that reviews patient care). The committee records of a covered committee are not available by discovery procedures to a party with adverse interest, and its individual members cannot be sued for their actions or decisions. However, most of the statutes provide immunity only if committee membership is made up of a particular group (primarily physicians) and if they act in good faith and without malice. Whether ethics committees would meet these statutory definitions in any one particular state is impossible to predict, without specific reference to the provisions of each state's statute and how the statute may have been interpreted in any prior litigation.

The only state that has, to date, established statutory protection for what appear to be ethics committees is Maryland.[8] In enacting its law with respect to "patient care advisory committees," the Maryland legislature specifically recognized the creation of committees that would "advise in cases involving life-threatening conditions—educate hospital personnel, patients, and patients' families concerning medical decision making—and review and recommend institutional policies and guidelines concerning the withholding of medical treatment." Maryland law specifically provides that the committee or any member "who gives advice in good faith may not be held liable in court for the advice given." It also grants confidentiality for the proceedings and deliberations and indicates that the advice itself should become part of the patient's medical record.

Committee membership in Maryland is statutorily defined to include a physician and a nurse not involved with the specific patient's care, a social worker, and the chief executive officer (CEO) of the facility or his or her designee. It also provides that the committee may additionally include members of the community and ethical advisors or clergy. However, it makes no mention of immunity for those who provide information to the committee or for any consultants that the committee involves in its deliberations.

Suits against the Ethics Committee or Its Members

In the unlikely event that a lawsuit is filed against an ethics committee, or against its individual members, naming them as defendants in a tort action, certain considerations arise regarding the defense of the action. Other considerations address who should assume responsibility for providing legal defense or paying a judgment.[9]

Hospital Employees

The actions of hospital employees appointed to the ethics committee by either the board of trustees, the CEO, or some other authority would be interpreted by the law as falling "within the scope of their employment." Provided they did not exceed that scope or did not willfully violate their responsibilities, their employer (the health care facility) would assume responsibility for their actions. In other words, the law sees the employer as responsible for the actions of its employees, as long as they act within the scope of their authority.

Most hospitals and health care facilities carry adequate insurance to cover their employees under such circumstances, that is, to pay any potential judgment rendered as well as the cost of defending the suit. This would be true for both public and private hospitals. It is critical, then, that the CEO or board of the facility ensure that employees who have been appointed to the ethics committee are adequately trained, thoughtful, prudent, and conscientious individuals who understand the extent of their responsibility and the seriousness of their mission. If either the ethics committee as a whole or its members exceed their authority, act in deliberate violation of hospital policy, or otherwise deviate from their mission, the hospital might deny responsibility for its/their actions. If their actions were egregious, the individuals themselves might be expected to defend the action and to pay defense costs as well as the judgment, if any.

Community Members

The same rules do not apply to community members who "volunteer" or are appointed to their position and who are not hospital employees. In such a situation, the hospital is not obligated vicariously, regardless of the volunteers' good faith, training, and so on. Under those circumstances, those who appoint public members of ethics committees should either seek umbrella coverage under the hospital's malpractice policy or provide these members with written assurance that the hospital will indemnify them against litigation, for payment of both a judgment and legal defense costs.

Physician Members

The rules are also different for physician members of the ethics committee. It would be advisable to specify the participation of physicians (employees) on the ethics committee in their list of clinical privileges, and therefore within the scope of their authority, so that, in the event a suit is filed, they would be adequately covered by the hospital's (employer's) malpractice policy.

However, independent, privately practicing physicians are not hospital employees. These physicians would have to look to their own individual malpractice policies for coverage relating to ethics committee activities. Because such circumstances have not arisen to date, it is impossible to predict how a malpractice insurance carrier would respond to this situation. If the policy included coverage for normal hospital committee activities, the physician is very likely to be covered. If the institution where that physician had clinical privileges provided coverage for all its medical staff for their normal hospital committee activities, this resource for coverage might be available to private physician committee members who were sued in such a setting. (Most malpractice insurance policies are written in terms of defending the physician insured against claims of negligence, an unintentional tort. If a suit filed against the ethics committee, including its physician members, alleged such actions as approving or abetting a battery, a false imprisonment, or a breach of confidentiality, the insurer might claim nonresponsibility to defend the action on the grounds that these were willful torts, as opposed to nonwillful ones.)

Perhaps the best defense of the reasonable, careful, thoughtful ethics committee member would be that he or she acted in good faith, with due care, without malice, and in conformity with thoughtful procedures and thorough investigation of the facts, and that the committee's conclusions and recommendations were reasonably warranted. Hospitals should consider providing a letter for all new ethics committee members that states their understanding of the duties of the committee, their expectations of committee members, and a statement of their own obligations. A sample of such a letter is provided in figure 9-1.

Conclusion

The criticism may be raised that ethics committee members are practicing law without a license when talking about legal requirements. Perhaps the best way to avoid this pitfall is for members to begin any discussion of the law with a disclaimer, stating in essence: "I am not an attorney and am not offering you legal advice. What I can do is tell you what I know about the statutes, their legislative history, the court holdings, any relevant government regulations, and the interrelationship of these. If you have a legal question, you should seek advice from your or the hospital's attorney."

There is potential for liability exposure in any action undertaken by a professional in the setting of health care delivery. Participation in the deliberations and actions of an ethics committee is no exception, despite the novelty of this particular arena and the "high-minded purpose" with which the committee undertakes its responsibility.

Chief executive officers and ethics committee members can best allay their fears about potential legal liability by ensuring the following (based on Staubach's suggestions):[10]

1. Careful development of the ethics committee's charge and mission
2. Thoughtful selection of the members
3. Continuing education of the members
4. Familiarity with the particulars of federal and state law (both legislation and case law)
5. Appropriate policies, protocols, guidelines, and documentation addressing the ethics committee's legal status and the hospital's obligations to its members

Figure 9-1. Sample Letter to New and Reappointed Members

The following is a sample of the letter that institutions might send to committee members either at the time they become members or each time they are reappointed.

Dear Committee Member:

May I take this opportunity, as the CEO of _____ hospital, to welcome you to service on our Bioethics Committee. The Board of Trustees and I, together with our entire staff and patient population, appreciate your willingness to volunteer your time, your expertise, and your concern to the mission of this facility.

As part of our commitment to assist you in this role, please be assured that we will provide you a period of orientation so that you may become familiar with the committee's charge and activities, as well as copies of the facility's mission statement, the ethics committee's mission statement, and a manual containing all relevant policies, procedures, and protocols of the facility and the ethics committee. These should be maintained in a confidential manner, for your information only, to be used solely in connection with your participation in the activities of the ethics committee. Following the completion of your tenure on this committee, we would expect you to return these materials to the facility.

As part of your service on this committee, you are expected to maintain the privacy and confidentiality of the patients, and to adhere to the protocols, policies, and procedures of the facility and of the ethics committee in its particular activities.

Ethics committee members are expected to be prudent, conscientious, and thorough in their approach to ethical problems as they are presented to the committee and discussed by committee members, focusing on the committee's goal of concern for the patient's best interests. You will not be expected to provide any information, guidance, or comments beyond those generated by your own personal experience, awareness, and knowledge. Certainly, you will not be expected or required to offer opinions beyond the scope of your own familiarity.

After consultation with hospital counsel and with the concurrence of the Board of Trustees, I can assure you that as long as the committee operates within its mission and appropriate functions within this facility as defined in its mission statement, this facility will provide legal counsel and cost of defense of any legal actions brought against you individually, as a committee member, for unintentional torts, arising out of your functions as a committee member. This facility will also cover the cost of any judgments that may be rendered against the committee as a whole or the members individually, as long as they operate within the scope of their authority. (The hospital may or may not be willing to cover the costs of counsel, legal defense, and judgment for willful torts as well [for example, battery, false imprisonment, violations of confidentiality or privacy, or defamation].)

6. Careful development of written protocols and procedures that the ethics committee will follow, particularly in case consultation
7. Comprehensive information gathering when conducting case review
8. Adequate time for thoughtful and thorough discussion of each case (if it cannot be done well, do not do it at all)
9. Appropriate and thorough documentation of the committee's conclusions, recommendations, and the data on which they are based in the committee's own record and summarized in the patient's medical record
10. Coverage of all committee members (including nonemployees) and their committee activities under the hospital's professional liability insurance policy or its general liability policy; or written assurance to public members that in the event of litigation, the facility will cover costs (defense and judgment) relating to their participation on the ethics committee

Exercises

1. If your committee has an attorney, ask members to write briefly what they expect that person to contribute to the committee in terms of his or her professional background. Give the responses to the attorney member and ask him or her to summarize and respond realistically to these expectations at the following meeting. For example, does the attorney find a match between his or her own and the committee members' expectations? If not, where is the mismatch? The purpose of this exercise is to come to clear agreement on what is and can be expected from a member with a particular expertise. The same exercise can

be carried out for other members (for example, the ethics consultant, the clinical ethicist, the administration representative, the clergy member).

2. There are data suggesting that far more negligence occurs in medical care than is litigated and that the nature of the relationship between professional and patient is correlated with the probability of a suit being filed in case of an adverse event. (Relationships characterized by psychological distance, unfamiliarity, or conflict are more likely to result in litigation.) In light of this, ask a patient who has filed a malpractice suit (not currently in litigation, of course) or has experienced an adverse event, a physician who has experienced a malpractice case, or an attorney who practices in this area to talk to the committee about the human dimensions of malpractice litigation. Consider the quality of the human relationships that your committee engenders in the course of prospective case review. What can the committee do to improve those relationships?

Notes and References

1. Personal communication (June 1992) with David Blake in which he argued that the distinction between law and ethics in bioethics is less clear-cut than is usually thought, largely because the case law has been developed in ways that are very similar to ethical analysis.

2. Meinhardt, R. The case for hospital lawyers on bioethics committees. *Ethical Currents* 22:4,8, 1990.

3. *Bouvia v. Superior Court, Glenchur et al.* (225 Cal Rptr., 297 [1986]).

4. Personal communication with Griffith Thomas, M.D., J.D., one of the attorneys in the case, Nov. 1991.

5. Merritt, A. The tort liability of hospital ethics committees. *Southern California Law Review* 1987;60:1239 (at 1272).

6. Cranford, R. E., Hester, F. A., and Ashley, B. Z. Institutional ethics committees: issues of confidentiality and immunity. *Law, Medicine and Healthcare* 13:52, Apr. 1985.

7. Siegler, M. Confidentiality in medicine: a decrepit concept. *New England Journal of Medicine* 307(24):1518, 1982.

8. Maryland statute section 19–372.

9. Staubach, S. What legal protection should a hospital provide, if any, to its ethics committee and individual members? *HEC Forum* 1(4):209, 1989.

10. Staubach.

10

Ethics Committee Relationships within the Institution: Special Concerns

In the early years of ethics committee development, most writers focused on the committee organization itself and its proposed functions. Now that some years of experience have accumulated, the need to clarify relationships between ethics committees and other entities (people and groups) is more apparent. This chapter looks at some of those relationships—with clinical ethicists, ethics consultants, domineering members, former members, former chairpersons, and other hospital committees. In addition, some thoughts are offered on terms of ethics committee membership and the advisability of permanent membership, a practice very different from that of many hospital committees.

How Ethics Committees Relate to Clinical Ethicists and Ethics Consultants

The number of people calling themselves ethicists seems to be increasing dramatically. In recent years, summer institutes and graduate degree programs in bioethics have flourished, resulting in many more people with some kind of formal training in bioethics. Because the word *ethicist* has no specific professional meaning, anyone who wishes to describe himself or herself as such can do so; and it is an accurate or successful description as long as there are people around who believe in the appellation.

In an effort to be more specific, this book distinguishes between two types of ethicist: the ethics consultant and the clinical ethicist. The *ethics consultant* is an individual who has received some special training in bioethics and has some responsibility for providing others with education on methods, trends, and phenomena in ethical and legal issues in health care. This person may be from a range of disciplines, although most frequently he or she is a philosopher, an attorney, or a clergy member. In more recent years, an ethics consultant is just as likely to be a physician or a nurse, because these professionals have become more actively involved in bioethics education programs. The *clinical ethicist* is an individual with the same kind of background as the ethics consultant but who has, in addition, formal responsibility for providing clinical ethics consultation, usually in the hospital. In short, the term *ethics consultant* is used here to describe an ethicist who does not have clinical responsibilities and the term *clinical ethicist* is used to describe an ethicist who has clinical responsibilities for assisting or directing the resolution of ethical problems in patient care. It is a distinction made in terms of *where* they work; both their qualifications and their relationship to the ethics committee may be the same.

The relationships of ethics committees with ethics consultants and clinical ethicists are complex, both historically and practically. These relationships may be supportive or conflict ridden. Those who had been involved in the field of bioethics for many years were among the first to help create ethics committees in the hospitals with which they were affiliated.

In some cases, they were and continue to be the driving force behind the committees in the role of ethics consultant. In other cases, they took on the role of clinical ethicist either in alliance with or in addition to their committee relationship. Sometimes the committees served a kind of apprenticeship with the ethicist and then took off on their own fledgling wings, with the ethicist as a continuing member. In some institutions, and more recently, ethicists have been hired and enjoined to create, as one of their charges, an ethics committee. Sometimes these ethicists have separate responsibilities for clinical consultation, sometimes they do not. However, this relationship evolved and whatever form it took, it is certainly a critical one for the ethics committee.

Clinical Ethicists

The relationship between the clinical ethicist and the ethics committee is usually greatly affected by how each came to be part of the institution. To the extent that there is conflict between the two, its source is most often centered on the consultation activity. First, ethics committees may be frozen out of the consultation activity because they do not function as efficiently as a single individual does. Second, a conflict of interest occurs if the clinical ethicist charges for consultations, that is, if he or she personally profits or if the hospital profits by having the clinical ethicist conduct the consultation rather than having the committee do so. There are no data on the number of clinical ethicists who charge for their services, nor on whether these individuals are also members of ethics committees.

Studies in the Literature

Data on clinical ethicists and ethics committees are very minimal. Fletcher and colleagues sent surveys to all "ethics consultants" (their term) who attended a 1985 conference on ethics consultation.[1] Thirty-eight individuals responded to a questionnaire whose questions primarily addressed the nature of their consultation activities. In addition, these clinical ethicists were asked whether their hospital had an ethics committee, whether they were a member of that committee, whether they chaired that committee, and whether there was some relationship between the ethics committee and their consultation activities. Only one-third of the respondents reported serving on the hospital ethics committee and the majority of those were not chairpersons. The report of this survey does not specify the number of institutions that had ethics committees, but presumably, if there was an ethics committee, the clinical ethicist was a member. If only one-third of these clinical ethicists were at institutions that had ethics committees, at the very least it certainly suggests that in 1985, clinical ethicists were not highly committed to the creation of ethics committees as either an extension of their own mission or groups with whom they could work collaboratively.

In a recent book in which 12 clinical ethicists at different institutions describe how they do "ethics at the bedside," only two of them specifically describe significant involvement of the ethics committee in the case consultation as it unfolds.[2] Four others invited one or two ethics committee members to observe or participate in the process, but this involvement appears to have been rather peripheral, with the ethicist organizing, controlling, and taking responsibility for the consultation. The remaining six authors either do not mention ethics committees at all or acknowledge that they chose not to involve committee members in the consultation. Although this book clearly is not intended to either capture typical consultations or describe the range of consultation methods, it suggests that clinical ethicists typically operate independently of the ethics committee.

Some ethicists have said that they describe all cases they have been involved in to the ethics committee as soon as possible (that is, at the following meeting). Others conduct their case consultation practice as an entirely separate activity to which the ethics committee is not privy. When both the clinical ethicist and the ethics committee are in the consultation business, there is always the risk of the medical staff shopping for the recommendations or suggestions they like best, and of both being consulted without the other's knowledge (and, in at least one case we know of, of receiving different recommendations).

In some institutions, the clinical ethicist works cooperatively with two or three members of the committee as a consultation team, thus providing perhaps the best melding of clinical ethicist and ethics committee.[3] This is most satisfactory (although more difficult), because it not only ensures adequate expertise (assuming the clinical ethicist is expert) but also preserves the virtues of at least some multidisciplinarity. It also sends the message that an ethicist alone is not sufficient to address ethical problems in patient care, that more than "expertise" is needed. However, this collaboration is difficult to achieve unless the clinical ethicist is particularly good at fostering a team approach. In the ordinary course of events, the clinical ethicist has more knowledge about bioethics and more time to devote to consultation activities than his or her clinician colleagues. Thus, it is easier to develop a leader–follower style of consultation than a genuine team or collegial approach.

The disagreement as to how clinical ethicists and committees should relate is succinctly demonstrated by two articles, each written by an internist who functions as a clinical ethicist in Illinois. Eric Loewy, a physician/clinical ethicist at the University of Illinois College of Medicine, in Peoria, has written of both his own experience in working with ethics committees and the possible relationship the clinical ethicist might have with the committee.[4] John LaPuma, a physician/clinical ethicist at Lutheran General Hospital, in Park Ridge, Illinois, also has addressed the topic of the relationship between clinical ethicist and ethics committee, although his writing does not reveal direct experience with these committees. It is notable that both Loewy and LaPuma also have appointments at the University of Chicago, whose medical ethics program has tended to endorse not only a strong preference for clinical ethicists over ethics committees, but also a preference for physicians as clinical ethicists over individuals from other disciplines.

Loewy and LaPuma have completely different views of how ethics committees and clinical ethicists should relate to one another, although both believe that the work of both entities can be complementary. LaPuma and Toulmin have strongly argued that complementarity means that clinical ethics consultants should do consultation, whereas ethics committees should focus on policy making.[5] Loewy, on the other hand, suggests that ethics committees should be available for consultation in those cases when the health care team does not wish to have the clinical ethicist involved (especially, he says, when there is only one such consultant in the hospital), when the physician responsible for the patient's care is unwilling to request a consultation, and when the clinical ethicist alone is unable to resolve the problem. In addition, he suggests that the committee "can serve as a critical audit committee for the retrospective review of cases seen by the consultant." He believes that such a review function serves all concerned: "When the committee reviews the judgments made by the ethics consultant, it can help educate the consultant just as the trained ethics consultant can, at times, help educate the committee."[6]

Although Loewy is clearly more sympathetic to a close involvement with the ethics committee, the ability to manage such involvement may be very much a matter of personality or timing. The clinical ethicist who is hired independently of the existence or creation of an ethics committee may have very little commitment to a close relationship and a diminished chance of creating such a relationship if the clinical ethicist is seen as impinging on the ethics committee's territory; the clinical ethicist whose task is to create the ethics committee may have a much greater commitment to both the committee's existence and its involvement in case review.

Making the Relationship Work

It is clear from the works of these clinical ethicists as well as from the writings of others[7] that some clinical ethicists relate more closely to ethics committees than do others. Thus, if institutions with one entity are considering having the other, a question they may want to ask themselves is: What relationship do we want the two to have? Are they to be separate but equal? Is one to subsume the other? If so, which is to be the "arm," as Fletcher states it, and which is to be the body? It seems likely that a clinical ethicist whose time is devoted to bioethics is more likely to control the committee than the reverse. If the institution's goal is for both the clinical ethicist and the ethics committee to support a common goal of heightened attention to ethical issues, it might consider involving the ethics committee in the decision to hire a clinical ethicist and even in his or her selection (at least as an interviewer of candidates). Moreover, the institution should insist that candidates for a clinical ethicist position describe how they plan to work cooperatively with the ethics committee.

Institutions also might want to consider a longer-term plan. For example, they might recognize someone within their institution who has a strong commitment to the institution's ethics committee and help that individual pursue more specialized education in anticipation of the time that the institution chooses to hire a clinical ethicist. That role can then be filled by a previously designated committee member who understands how the committee works and who will be able to work with it.

Ethics committees and clinical ethicists need not be in conflict. However, if more clinical ethicists are to be hired in the future, as some have suggested, it is likely that the ethics committee will precede the hiring of the clinical ethicist. That factor is likely to make that relationship more difficult, particularly if the clinical ethicist sees his or her position as one of primarily providing clinical case consultation, with assistance to or involvement with the ethics committee as a secondary or incidental aspect of the job.

Ethics Consultants

In addition to clinical ethicists, many committees have relationships with ethics consultants who are not clinical ethicists. These are individuals who may have studied bioethics extensively; who teach bioethics in undergraduate colleges, community colleges, nursing schools, medical schools, law schools, and so on; or who have degrees in bioethics but do not have any formal responsibility for addressing ethical issues in the clinical setting. Thus, the ethics consultant does not present the potential for conflict of interest that the clinical ethicist does. He or she is included or excluded at the committee's will. Ethics consultants often take on responsibility for educating the ethics committee but, most frequently, do not chair the committee. Typically, the ethics consultant usually comes from outside the medical setting, although perhaps not from very far outside (for example, the hospital's corporate office or a nearby university or college sometimes formally connected with the hospital).

Potential Source of Conflict

The primary source of conflict between the ethics consultant and the ethics committee is the tendency for the consultant to dominate the committee, even if he or she is not its chairperson. The consultant's broader knowledge of the field may be seen by members as conclusive, stifling discussion. That is particularly the case if the ethics "expert" has no particular commitment to empowering the committee through education. However, in an ethics committee that has been well educated from the beginning, committee style and the kinds of issues that committees address seem to be more a function of the interests and personalities of individual committee members than of the preferences of an ethics consultant. For example, the consultant's interests in evaluation are seldom shared by ethics committee members. His or her sense of the cutting-edge issues often does not reflect the interests and experiences of committee members. Except in committees that do many consultations (a distinct minority), most of the discussion topics are raised by committee members themselves. Members tend to look to the ethics consultant not for answers but for information about practices elsewhere, legal cases, and so forth.

At the formation stage of the committee (perhaps the first year), members rely on the ethics consultant for information, resources, general themes, and trends. After that, they probably are just as content to plunge on alone, although over time they may feel rather isolated from the larger ethics committee movement if they do not maintain a relationship with someone who has a professional interest in and commitment to the field, or if some members do not commit themselves to more reading, conference attending, and networking than is typical of the average committee member.

The ethics consultant may have no background in the clinical setting. Such an individual's desire or tendency to dominate committee views is likely to be counterbalanced by the clinical experience of the committee members. In effect, the ethics consultant may know how things are supposed to be, but not how they really are. This difference usually helps keep everyone reasonably humble about moving to solutions for the problem of the day. For example, consider the following scenario in which a committee was considering the appropriate way to address DNR orders for a patient who lacked capacity and had no family or other surrogate, and for whom the attending physician considered a DNR order appropriate.

The ethics consultant suggested court appointment of a temporary conservator. However, the clinicians on the committee knew their colleagues would not be inclined to do that because of the extra work involved and the length of time required to achieve their goal. The ethics consultant then suggested review by a second physician. The clinicians in turn pointed out that it is unlikely that any physician would approach someone likely to disagree with his or her judgment on this point. (In this hospital, it was not possible for the ethics committee itself to review the decision.)

The ethics consultant and the clinicians on the committee compromised by requiring the attending physician to document in detail the reasons for judging that resuscitation was not in this particular patient's best interest. In this case, the ethics consultant understood the theoretically correct approach to the case, but did not truly understand the environment in which the case arose nor the impact of that environment on decision making.

Identification of the Consultant's Role

As mentioned earlier, the ethics consultant often takes on the role of educator. In this capacity, he or she serves as a link to the larger bioethics and ethics committee movements (keeping members informed of new bioethics research and legal cases; of discussions in the literature of ethics committee roles and methodologies; and of the larger field of which ethics committees are a part), as a constructive critic of the committee's process, and as a gentle force to keep the committee focused on service to the hospital community rather than to its own interests exclusively. The committee can help the consultant by clearly communicating both what the members do and do not find helpful and how much participation by the ethics consultant is desired. Most consultants are involved with more than one ethics committee and find that different committees want different things from them. However, the committee that expects the consultant to do all the work while its other members are willing only to attend the meetings has in fact relinquished its responsibilities to the consultant. The committee that says "we want you to be an equal member of this committee, with an equal right of participation and equal expectations of contribution" is clear about what it wants. The committee that expects educational input and advice only when the consultant is asked also is clear about a legitimate role for the ethics consultant. But most committees never consciously address the role of the ethics consultant. Thus, it is left to the consultant to constantly judge how much and how little to offer and do. Committees that have ethics consultants might make better use of them if they thought more directly about what they want from them.

Physician Dominance of Committees

Because hospitals have a hierarchical structure, with physicians at or near the top, physician dominance of ethics committees has consistently been a problem. Some committees are dominated by a single physician, which is more a problem of effective leadership (see chapter 4 on meetings) than of physician dominance as a general issue. On many committees, however, physicians both numerically dominate the group and vocally dominate discussions. Such committees are likely to demonstrate a continuing lack of genuine interdisciplinary achievement. Without interdisciplinarity, the committee cannot truly be called an ethics committee. It may be a committee about doctors' solutions to their ethical problems in the same way that a nursing ethics committee is about nurses' solutions to their ethical problems, but it has not yet been born as an interdisciplinary ethics committee.

Some physicians complain that nurses and other allied health professionals either are too timid to participate or do not understand physicians' ethical (and legal) problems. Although physicians are seldom reluctant to participate in ethics committee discussions (whereas some nurses and allied health professionals are), everyone has plenty to learn, and one of the first things to be learned is how to create an environment in which everyone's contributions are welcome. If members have nothing to contribute, the committee may need to reconsider the manner in which it selects members. It is easy to find a dozen people in the hospital who have a great deal to contribute to the discussion of ethical issues in patient care. Learning to listen to others is the first step. If some members need to learn more, it is a virtue that there are others on the committee who are in a position to help them do that.

Achieving interdisciplinarity is not easy. It is not enough to put 15 people from different disciplines in a room for an hour or two and let each have a turn at talking. To achieve inter-disciplinarity requires the creation of a group whose members respect one another, have the ability to acquire both listening and "translation" skills (the ability and willingness to trans-late the technical words, jargon, and conceptual approaches unique to one discipline into a language that can be understood by people from other disciplines) and are willing to adhere to the group process. Even though physicians may numerically dominate the committee, they need not and should not dominate the nature of its work. Physicians have been socialized to see themselves as the "captain of the ship," and this often makes it difficult for them to work collegially with nonphysicians. Because physicians as a group still tend to be male and nonphysicians in the health care system tend to be female, there also is an overlay of gender problems in the issue of physician dominance.

There is an increasing body of work that attempts to look at how men and women differ in the ways they relate to their work, the world, and each other. One resource that may be particularly helpful to ethics committee members is Deborah Tannen's *You Just Don't Under-stand,*[8] which focuses on the differences between male and female communication styles. Because much of what makes an ethics committee successful depends on its members being able to discuss with each other their different perspectives and values, members would benefit from a sensitivity to these kinds of issues.

Other ways that physician dominance can be minimized include ensuring that:

- Nurses, social workers, and clergy selected for committee membership are articulate individuals in groups.
- Subcommittees are chaired by members other than physicians.
- The right to vote is extended to all members of the committee (not just physicians, as is required by some medical staff rules).
- Meetings begin when a quorum of *members* is present, not a quorum of *physician members*.
- Education programs designed for physicians include as presenters nonphysician members of the committee.
- Education on new policies is conducted for physicians, not just for nurses.
- First names, not titles, are used for all members.

The committee's multidisciplinarity must be taken seriously if the committee is to present the kind of collegial relationship and problem solving that is different from the customary hospital model.

As a practical matter, if the committee has a good balance of members who are willing to participate but physicians still dominate the meeting, the chairperson should be encouraged to intervene in the process. For example, the discussion of a topic could begin by the chair-person's suggestion that each person in turn give a quick picture of how he or she views the major problem. Or, later in the discussion, the chairperson could suggest taking the tem-perature of the group by asking the members to say quickly where they find themselves at that point. Such democratizing process moves can help mitigate domination. Finally, meetings can conclude with a quick written evaluation that includes a question on whether everyone felt that he or she was able to be heard. Reviewing the feedback at the next meeting makes this issue explicit and, over time, can change behaviors. This kind of informal evaluation can be used for other committee process problems as well. However, it is seldom used — probably because it seems too formal for a meeting. But if people are willing to come to a meeting, they should be willing to say why it was or was not worth their time. Regular feedback *can* make a difference.

Membership Terms

As committees find themselves celebrating eighth and tenth or more anniversaries, it is becoming apparent to them that some way of inviting more people to experience committee membership is essential. The following subsections offer ideas on how to accomplish this.

Rotating Members

Many committees have chosen to rotate a portion of their membership every year (for example, one-half or one-third of the members are replaced each year by new members). Obviously, this can be a blessing for those committees who got the wrong members in the first place. For those committees who were fortunate enough to get committed and contributing members, rotating membership frequently creates problems. It takes at least five or six years for an ethics committee to develop expertise, a common memory, a sense of humility, an appropriate level of frustration tolerance, and an appropriate level of hope for change. The advantage of shorter terms is that more individuals are exposed to the discussion of ethical issues. The disadvantage is that no one develops very much sophistication on method, complexity of the issues, or even complexity of the group to which he or she belongs.

A Hybrid of Core and Rotating Members

Some committees are now considering a hybrid form of committee membership in which approximately half the members will be "core" or ex officio members[9] assigned to the committee for as long as they choose and the remainder will be rotating members who participate on the committee for three or four years. This solution attempts to both preserve the committee's experience, historical memory, and group identification, and expose the committee's work to more individuals throughout the institution.

Problems in determining who will be core members (and who will make that determination) are considerable, running as they do into our cultural ideals of a democratic process in which everyone has equal opportunity to participate. It is imaginable that a committee that has been in existence for a number of years with a fairly steady membership could actually determine through a voting consensus those members whom it believes to be most essential to its ongoing functioning. It is also imaginable that such a process, if not carefully handled, could result in considerable harm to the committee's sense of itself.

Other problems include selection of the committee chairperson (whether he or she should be a core member); selection of new core members should one leave; and division of labor between core members and rotating members. The creation of a two-tier structure is worrisome in a committee struggling to overcome hierarchy problems. Furthermore, such a two-tier committee might intensify the idea that ethics is a matter of special expertise and not a matter for everyone.

An alternative way to achieve this same goal might be to reappoint any member who has made particularly strong contributions during his or her initial period of membership. This is an attractive solution unless such an individual is from a discipline that has low representation on the committee. For example, many committees have only one "social worker slot." If the member from that discipline is perennially reappointed, no other social worker will have the opportunity to serve on the committee. Core membership would eliminate this problem because the range of membership selection would be based on the open committee positions and not on the core ones. In addition, decisions about reappointment could be as difficult as those about selection of core members, and they would have to be made frequently rather than rarely.

Permanent Members

Another alternative is for the committee to keep all its members indefinitely; that is, membership is permanent as long as the member wishes to stay and participates. If this method is chosen, the committee will need to involve other hospital personnel in ways other than their being the subject of the committee's education efforts. Frequently, the committee will need to find ways of collaborating with other individuals. For example, they may be invited to educate the committee itself, they may be asked to be members of ad hoc committees when they have special expertise that is needed, and so forth. Permanent membership can be a viable way of organizing a committee, but it runs the risk of making the committee appear to be the "owner" of ethics and not the facilitator of ethical resolution.

Continuity with Former Members

If ethics committees are to succeed in the long run, they must be able to maintain continuity with their most experienced and committed members without becoming a closed group. Sometimes it seems that the field changes daily with new issues and new ideas on how best to function in the institutional setting during a tumultuous time for health care. The strength of the committee must be preserved by ensuring that knowledgeable and skilled members continue to work together to further the committee's mission. Committees are already trying to create relationships with former members. Some methods they are or could be using to preserve these relationships include:

- Appointing interested former committee members to participate on subcommittees
- Inviting former members to be guests at meetings
- Naming former members as alternate committee members
- Including former members on core consultation teams
- Inviting former members to sit in on meetings to offer informal evaluations of the committee process
- Having former members (especially chairpersons) meet with steering committees to help plan the future of the committee

Although these are productive ways to maintain continuity with former members, they may be too informal for ensuring the committee's continuity and strength. A more formal method of ensuring continuity might include the creation of a permanent advisory committee of former members who would have specific tasks, such as evaluation of the committee's overall well-being, liaison with the hospital community, orientation of new members, and so on.

The Role of Former Chairpersons

Many ethics committees have now been in existence long enough to have experienced not only rotation of several members off the committee, but also replacement of the chairpersons. Ethics committees usually bear the imprint of their chairpersons, from the standpoint of procedure, involvement of committee members, emphases on particular aspects of committee work, and case review procedures. New chairpersons do not always proceed in the same manner as their predecessors, which has the potential for creating a disconcerting and disappointing experience for ex-chairpersons who continue to be members of the committee after their term has come to an end. Their frustration can become overwhelming, particularly when they see the child they have loved and nurtured through a troubled infancy and adolescence now "go astray" under the guidance of another. An ex-chairperson's disappointment may even be coupled with a sense of failure, particularly if the ex-chairperson has taken pains to train his or her successor.

It might be advisable for ex-chairpersons who find themselves in this position to seek a new role, perhaps as mentor for new or potential committee members during their early educational phase, to help "bring them up to speed" with longer-standing committee members. Or, in an auxiliary role, they might wish to run small educational projects such as brown-bag lunches, discussion groups, and so forth for particular services, ward groups, house officers, and medical students throughout the facility.

After a period of time off the committee, ex-chairpersons, and perhaps even ex-members, might be reappointed to the committee. It is wasteful to spend a great deal of time and effort educating committee members, letting them feel comfortable in all aspects of committee function, and turning them into knowledgeable, valuable resources for the institution as a whole only to dismiss them from the committee after their term of office has been completed. They can be used as a continuing educational resource within their own service or discipline to help raise the level of ethical familiarity and awareness throughout the institution and to anticipate those situations where ethical dilemmas might arise in the future. Additionally, they may be used as a resource for staff education in compliance with the Patient Self-Determination Act and as a resource to help patients and their families, as well as the larger hospital community, learn more about advance directives and rights to consent to and refuse treatment as part of the educational effort required by the act.

If an outgoing chairperson has established a particular style in the conduct of ethics committee meetings, a new chairperson may prove a disappointment to committee members who have become accustomed to the "old way" of doing things. They may find it difficult to adjust to a new chairperson, whose emphasis and approach may be very different. It is important to acknowledge these transitions, not only by thanking the former chairperson for his or her leadership and guidance but also by devoting a meeting or a significant portion of a meeting at the time of the transition to a discussion of the achievements of the past year and the hopes and expectations for the next year under the new chairperson's leadership. One retiring chairperson chose to evaluate the committee's progress during his leadership and also to discuss what he saw as his failures or weaknesses. This offered committee members an opportunity to discuss their feelings about what was and was not working—a discussion that the incoming chairperson could put to good use. Such a transition discussion can heighten the sense of collegiality that makes ethics committee work so rewarding.

Any former chairperson has a difficult role. In some ways, the ex-chairperson may be something of an elder statesman, but in other ways, he or she may be seen as a barrier to change or progress. Former chairpersons should use all their political skills and lingering authority to enhance the committee's well-being. This may mean sacrificing their personal views about the best way to do things or it may mean risking an accusation of interference. As in the care of a patient, careful consideration of where the committee's best interests lie may lead to great uncertainty. And, again as in the care of the patient, a decision must be made about whether to do something.

For example, consider the situation of an ex-committee chairperson who reports that members of the committee who continued on under the leadership of the new chairperson have advised him that the new chairperson does all case consultation by himself, without involving the subcommittee for case review, which had been the method of performing this task under the ex-chairperson's leadership. Committee members are frustrated and do not know how to approach the new chairperson with their concerns but find comfort in telling the former chairperson—which only increases his disappointment and frustration. Should the former chairperson in this situation discuss the issue with the new chairperson? Should he counsel the committee members to bring the issue to the attention of the new chairperson? Should he coach them in strategies to achieve their goal? Should he wash his hands of the whole matter as no longer being his problem?

What role the former chairperson plays will of course depend on many issues specific to the setting, but committees need to consider the possibilities carefully. This is an issue that ethics committee networks might want to address by bringing together a number of former chairpersons to discuss their experiences and their relationship with their ethics committee.

Ethics Committees and Other Institutional Committees

The Joint Commission on Accreditation of Healthcare Organizations' (JCAHO's) *Accreditation Manual for Hospitals* defines a variety of functions and activities that JCAHO reviews in its member hospitals on a regular basis. For the first time, the 1991 manual refers to ethical concerns and ethics committees under Standard NC.3.[10] This standard requires that nursing policies and procedures include internal review for information on "ethical and legal concerns" (NC.3.1.2.5.2). In addition, it requires that "nursing staff members have a defined mechanism for addressing ethical issues in patient care, and that when the hospital has an ethics committee or other defined structures for addressing ethical issues in patient care, nursing staff members participate" (NC.3.2). The manual goes further (RI.1.1.6.1) by requiring that organizations have "in place a mechanism(s) for the consideration of ethical issues arising in the care of patients and to provide education to caregivers and patients on ethical issues in health care." Although ethics committees have not been mandated by the JCAHO, they have been given significant recognition by this mention.

For purposes of smooth operation, the JCAHO manual specifies that the hospital staff should be organized to accomplish its required functions. For the most part, these functions are accomplished by many specific committees or groups. These groups provide many mechanisms for dealing with issues that are clearly ethical but beyond the scope of the ethics committee. The ethics committee should complement these groups, not substitute for them or interfere with their work. If they are not functioning properly, the ethics committee can play a role in alerting the proper authorities, making suggestions for possible resolutions, and so on. But the ethics committee should be cognizant of the fact that, despite its name, it is not the only entity in the hospital responsible for and capable of dealing with ethical issues.

Hospital committee membership is primarily representational. For example, the Medical Records Committee may include representatives from the various sections or services of the medical staff, as well as from nursing, pharmacy, and whatever other clinical services are required or permitted to make entries into the patient's medical record. Members of the ethics committee, on the other hand, may not be as representational of a particular service, section, or department but, instead, are selected on the basis of each individual's interests, abilities, background, education, dedication, and willingness to commit substantial time to both learning and service. The committee's charge, in terms of its definition in the bylaws, is critical in determining exactly what its responsibilities are and how it may interpret its role.

For example, if the ethics committee has been established merely because "every other hospital in the city has one," its annual report to the medical staff may consist only of a description of its educational activities, a list of the policies it has reviewed and/or recommended for consideration by the medical staff, a brief outline of the number of case reviews it has performed, and a list of the committee members. However, if the committee's charge is to be the "ethical conscience of the institution," the committee's interpretation of its role may be entirely different and would involve relationships with other hospital committees. It might be hoped that in the memorandum establishing the ethics committee, there is specific mention of the committee's responsibilities in patient care as a whole within the institution (giving the committee greater scope) and in reporting its findings and recommendations.

Following are some examples of committee roles and their relationships to other committees:

- The ethics committee at hospital A has appointed a subcommittee that regularly reviews a specific percentage of all deaths or discharges in cases where a DNR order has been written to determine the extent of compliance with the facility's DNR policy. This retrospective review is reported at committee meetings on a bimonthly basis and a summary, which includes the service where the patient was admitted but does not include patient or physician names, is sent to the executive committee of the medical staff on a regular basis.

One committee member suggested that perhaps, because this had to do with medical records, a copy of that report should also be submitted to the medical records review committee. After thorough discussion by the committee members in attendance, it was decided that such action would be inappropriate because the committee had no reporting responsibilities to the medical records review committee. Accordingly, the reports were continued only to the executive committee for its decision and action with respect to referral to the medical records review committee. On further questioning, committee members felt they would be overstepping their authority in reporting their findings to a group other than the medical staff or its executive committee.

- The ethics committee in another hospital performed concurrent medical record reviews to determine how well physicians were complying with hospital policy regarding the writing of DNR orders prior to instituting an educational effort throughout the institution directed at increasing compliance with the policy. In this case, too, one member suggested that perhaps a report should be sent to the medical records review committee. In this case as well, the committee voted down that suggestion as not being appropriate in view of the purpose for which the concurrent review was undertaken, that is, to determine the extent of the educational effort needed with respect to the hospital policy.

- After reviewing medical records retrospectively, the ethics committee in a third hospital sent its findings regarding compliance to the quality assurance committee of the service that was deficient in recording DNR orders consistent with hospital policy requirements. In that case, it was suggested that the service in question might wish to use compliance with the documentation requirements of the DNR policy as one of its quality assurance monitors in further QA reviews.

  The appropriateness of such a referral might be questioned, because the ethics committee charge contained no reference to its authority to refer its findings to other hospital committees or services regarding compliance with facility policy. However, the committee was particularly concerned about two physicians who appeared to routinely write DNR orders without patient/surrogate knowledge or consent.

- After a flurry of case consultations brought by members of the nursing staff on the psychiatric ward of an acute care hospital, the ethics committee became aware that certain medications were being used inappropriately on that service. Committee members agonized over whether these improprieties in medication administration should be reported to the pharmacy and therapeutics committee, to the drug utilization review committee, or the chairperson of the particular department.

  After determining that other patients would be at significant risk if prior practices were to be continued, the chairperson of the ethics committee and two other members met informally with the chairperson of the department and then with the chief of staff, without documenting their concerns in their minutes. This led to a full-blown peer review investigation generated by the chief of staff. To its credit, the committee had kept accurate and complete records regarding its review of the cases to adequately defend against allegations of malice and lack of good faith raised by the accused physicians. The thorough documentation and reporting through the chain of command to the chief of staff and the executive committee were critical elements. It would have been very different had the ethics committee decided on its own to report to a peer review group or the credentials and privileges committee.

- An ethics committee in a large teaching hospital became aware that any time a patient or patient surrogate in the coronary care unit (CCU) requested that a DNR order be placed in the chart, the patient was automatically transferred to a lower level of care. This became known after family members requested ethics committee consultation to determine why what appeared to them to be appropriate care was being denied to the patient.

  After review of the situation, and discussion with the chief of CCU, the ethics committee determined that its best course was to institute an intensive educational effort for all the members of the medical staff who admitted patients to the CCU, as well as the nursing staff there, to develop a consistent approach to this type of patient. When the issue of possible referral to the utilization review (UR) committee was made, the ethics committee voted against it in favor of waiting to see how successful its educational efforts were. Subsequently, there appeared to be a softening of the prior consistently hard-line approach to such requests by patients, and referral to the UR committee was deemed unnecessary.

The ethics committee should become familiar with the political relationships within the facility as a whole. If it is the perception of the medical staff that the ethics committee considers itself a self-appointed watchdog or guardian angel over all hospital activities, the committee's position within the institution may be in jeopardy and its credibility, if not its very existence, may be destroyed. This is not to advocate a "go-along-to-get-along" policy by the ethics committee but, rather, a more basic approach to reexamining the nature of its real responsibilities in terms of promoting the patient's best interests. If the medical staff as a whole becomes alienated from the committee, the committee will not have accomplished any of its goals and, as noted above, may jeopardize its very existence.

For example, consider the following dilemma. The ethics committee becomes aware of a physician on the staff, well connected politically and well established within the hierarchy of the institution, who continues to be in direct and conscious violation of hospital policy and patients' legal rights by continuing treatment for patients who have stated they no longer want such treatment. After several carefully written and prudent entries by the ethics committee in the medical records of the patients involved and requests by various nurses to review the situation (ignored by the physician), it is clear to the committee that the physician in question has no intention of changing his approach or his course of action in such cases; that is, he is committed to continuing ventilatory support to patients who have requested that such support be withdrawn. The committee invites the physician to attend one of its meetings to discuss patients' rights, but he refuses to attend.

How is this committee to proceed? The facility's legal counsel might be contacted, particularly because the facility stands at great legal risk in terms of exposure to liability for violation of the patient's rights, lack of informed consent, and potential allegations of battery, to name just a few. The physician is obviously in violation of the facility's policy. Just how far a committee should go under circumstances such as these remains a question. The committee could reasonably take the issue through the usual chain of command, where the next higher authority has responsibility for acting once it has received the information. Going public could result in a breach of confidentiality for all involved. These issues probably would be handled best in anticipation, that is, in drafting the ethics committee's charge or mission or in defining its own guidelines, protocols, or procedures. Being prepared for unusual cases such as these is the best way to avoid potential legal hazards in which everyone loses.

Institutional Review Boards

The hospital committee most like the ethics committee is the institutional review board (IRB). The IRBs were established in response to federal legislation, enacted following recommendations of the National Commission for the Protection of Human Subjects, which required that all institutions receiving research funding from the federal government establish a review board to oversee and review all research projects involving biomedical or behavioral study in order to ensure that they meet ethical standards, particularly as they affect the rights of potential subjects. These committees are multidisciplinary and include members of the lay public as well as the research community. In view of their legislative mandate, IRBs can make binding, formal decisions with respect to research. They also have the obligation to review consent forms, which patients must execute as part of entry into a research project. Although ethics committees have neither the mandate nor the authority to make formal or binding decisions, their involvement in ethical aspects of patient care is parallel to the IRB's. In some cases, it may even overlap.

For example, at one institution a researcher asked the ethics committee to review a particular situation before he brought it to the members of the IRB and the research committee as a whole. The researcher was evaluating cardiac medications for treatment of a particular disease entity. The research design of this project was such that it was a single-blind study. Before the complete number of research subjects had been entered into the protocol, the researcher realized that the treatment group fared uniformly well whereas the control group did very poorly. He wished to discontinue the study, because he could not in good conscience continue to enroll patients in the control group, feeling fairly certain that their outcome would be less than optimal. He asked the ethics committee's concurrence in approaching the IRB and the research committee for permission to discontinue the study, without prejudice.

In reviewing the matter with the researcher, the ethics committee questioned whether he had been biased in his selection of patients for the control group (as opposed to the treatment group). He assured the committee that he had selected patients on a random basis, the assignment decision actually having been made by his technician. He was then asked whether he thought patients would be harmed by continuing to be enrolled in the control group. He responded affirmatively. It was suggested that the researcher approach the IRB without any further ethics committee involvement. The ethics committee felt that it had discharged its responsibilities by helping the researcher to think through his evaluation of the ethical elements involved in the research project.

Another IRB requested that two protocols be referred to the ethics committee for review and analysis before the IRB considered approving their patient selection methods. One involved the use in a double-blind study of four possible drugs for the treatment of a neurological emergency. Following successful treatment of the acute condition, patients invited to participate would be given the drugs in random selection to determine which of the four was most effective and had the fewest side effects. However, because it was an emergency, patient consent could not be obtained *before* entry into the study. The IRB felt that it was inappropriate to treat a patient on a research protocol as part of an emergency situation and then obtain consent after the fact to continue in follow-up. Referral to the ethics committee was requested to help sort out this dilemma.

The second request involved a consent form for treatment of certain types of cancer using experimental drugs on a double-blind basis, whereas conventional therapy, with a high rate of success, would be withheld. The IRB was concerned that the consent form did not adequately spell out the fact that patients receiving the experimental drug would in essence be denying themselves the opportunity to be treated with acceptable conventional therapy, which had previously shown a high success rate. The IRB wanted the concurrence of the ethics committee to ensure that the patients' rights were not being inappropriately infringed upon.

This kind of close relationship between ethics committees and IRBs probably is the exception rather than the rule. Some IRBs may restrict themselves to such issues as adequacy of informed consent documents, and ask ethics committees for assistance on other issues with which they have less familiarity. Others may see research as the IRB's responsibility and patient care as the ethics committee's responsibility, and keep a sharp division between them.

However, because many of the concerns are similar and parallel, it may be appropriate for individuals on one committee (the IRB) to rotate subsequently to membership on the ethics committee or to sit on both committees, when both such committees exist within a particular facility. The issues to come before the committees may raise similar concerns and the cross-fertilization may be an extremely valuable asset to be encouraged and fostered. A member's participation on one certainly raises his or her level of awareness for issues that come before the other. If nothing else, the committees can be mutually supportive and perhaps participate in joint educational activities throughout the facility to help raise the level of concern among employees and staff with respect to ethical issues in patient care and research. They would then be fulfilling the mandate originally envisioned in the establishment of the President's Commission for the Study of Ethical Problems in Medicine and Biomedical and Behavioral Research.

Conclusion

Nurturing relationships with others in the institution—whether former members or other committees—may help prevent or reduce much of the isolation that ethics committees often feel. During the early years of their development, few committees had time for anything beyond a narrow understanding of their functions. However, over time, a fuller consideration of relationships to others becomes productive in helping convey the message that ethics is everyone's concern and not the private domain of the ethics committee.

Exercises

Committees might discuss the following questions, as appropriate to their setting:

1. Are members happy with the committee's relationship with the institution's clinical ethicist? Do they know what that relationship is?
2. Would the committee function better if it had an ethics consultant as a member?
3. Does the committee understand what is expected of the ethics consultant? Is that what is wanted? Does the committee's ethics consultant understand what the committee wants of him or her?
4. Would a clinical ethicist help achieve the committee's mission in the hospital?
5. Is there some member of the committee you would want to propose to the hospital administration as a potential clinical ethicist?
6. What do former committee members think of the ethics committee now that they are no longer members?
7. Would many people in the institution like to be on the ethics committee? Do they have a realistic opportunity of that happening?
8. Is the ethics committee getting stale as a result of having had the same members for too long?
9. In what capacity can the former chairpersons continue to contribute to the committee?
10. If a person has been a committee chairperson, what are the burdens and benefits of having him or her continue on as a member of the committee? Of preventing him or her from being a member?
11. Does this hospital have an IRB? Do committee members feel competent to discuss the ethical issues involved in research protocols? Should they?
12. Has the committee had cases in which it should have considered reporting information to other hospital committees? Should it report cases to other committees? If, for example, the committee repeatedly sees cases that demonstrate problems in continuity of care, does it have an obligation to deal with the systemic problems that lead to such discontinuity? How does it do it? Should the committee establish protocols?
13. What other institutional committees do ethics committee members sit on? Should the ethics committee request having formal liaison members with other committees?

Notes and References

1. Fletcher, J. C., Quist, N., and Jonsen, A. R., editors. A survey of ethics consultants: appendix. In: *Ethics Consultation in Health Care.* Ann Arbor, MI: Health Administration Press, 1989, p. 199.

2. Culver, C. M., editor. *Ethics at the Bedside.* Hanover, NH: University Press of New England, 1990.

3. Younger, S. I've changed my mind. In: C. M. Culver, editor. *Ethics at the Bedside.* Hanover, NH: University Press of New England, 1990, pp. 99–126. Younger shows this melding most effectively.

4. Loewy, E. H. Ethics consultation and ethics committees. *HEC Forum* 2(6):351–59, 1990.

5. La Puma, J., and Toulmin, S. E. Ethics committees and ethics consultants. *Archives of Internal Medicine* 149(5):1109–12, 1989, p. 356.

6. Loewy.

7. See, for example, Ruth Macklin's description of the ethics committee's involvement in cases in *Mortal Choices* (Boston: Houghton-Mifflin, 1987, pp. 224–30) and John Fletcher and colleagues' descriptions of their consultation service (an "arm" of the institutional ethics committee) in the article entitled Biomedical ethics and the ethics consultation service at the University of Virginia (*HEC Forum* 2(2):89–99, 1990).

8. Tannen, D. *You Just Don't Understand: Women and Men in Conversation.* New York City: Ballantine Books, 1990.

9. The ex officio membership is sometimes used for ethics consultants so that they are not rotated off the committee.

10. Joint Commission on Accreditation of Healthcare Organizations. *Accreditation Manual for Hospitals.* Oakbrook Terrace, IL: JCAHO, 1991.

11

Ethics Committees outside the Hospital: Long-Term Care and Community Care

It is estimated that although 60 percent of the hospitals in the United States have some kind of ethics committee or forum, only 8 to 10 percent of nursing homes have formed such groups.[1] Most of biomedical ethics and the agenda for ethics committees over the past 10 years has been established in acute care facilities and around acute care issues. Yet it is chronic illness, often accompanied by dementia and/or physical disability, that has become more common in the health care system. Health care is increasingly being delivered, and medical decisions are being made, outside hospital walls — in nursing homes, residential hospices, and patients' homes under the auspices of home care and hospice care. It is only natural that the prospect of replicating hospital ethics committees in these other environments would attract attention.

Some of the early long-term care committees responded to and focused on issues of life-sustaining technologies. One such committee at the Hebrew Home of Greater Washington (in Rockville, Maryland) was established in 1979 and throughout its 11-year existence the issue of feeding has persisted as the most troublesome topic.[2] A long-standing ethics committee in a religion-based extended care facility in Los Angeles had considerable difficulty with termination of treatment decisions because of its religious orientation.[3]

Whether as a result of religious affiliation or because of concerns about state regulation and sanctions, long-term care facilities have not kept up with the acute care hospitals in forgoing treatment decisions. The Patient Self-Determination Act (abbreviated as PSDA and effective as of December 1991) requires long-term care institutions receiving Medicare or Medicaid reimbursements to inform patients of their rights to consent to and refuse treatment and to complete advance directives such as durable powers of attorney for health care and living wills. In addition, the PSDA requires the facilities to document whether patients have advance directives and to inform patients of the facilities' own policies with respect to honoring patient preferences. As a result, nursing homes are being forced to catch up with some of the issues that hospitals have been addressing for the past decade.

It is likely that ethics committees will form in and for nursing homes to help meet the requirements of this federal act and that that will be the primary thrust of long-term care ethics committees for some time to come. Nevertheless, the issue of forgoing life-sustaining treatment, when compared to other ethical issues in long-term care, is relatively insignificant in frequency and impact, although its symbolic importance continues to be great. Moreover, administrators appear to perceive it as the central (and perhaps only) ethical problem they face in long-term care, failing to see that financial and personal life-style issues are perhaps more laden with ethical problems.[4]

To understand why life-sustaining treatment decisions may be of less practical importance and to determine how ethics committees are or can be helpful in long-term care settings, it is important to examine the differences between acute and chronic care and then to develop a list of ethics issues arising in the course of chronic care. It is also essential to appreciate the institutional, environmental, and provider constraints within which this care is delivered.

Ethics committees in acute care hospitals that are helping nursing homes start their own ethics committees need this information, but it is also important that nursing home staff appreciate how these differences alter the way in which ethics committees can be realized in extended care. It is not a simple or direct transplantation. Although concerns with patient well-being, patient autonomy, and multidisciplinary responses to problems remain the same, the following differences need to be considered:

- Physicians have much less contact with patients and staff in nursing homes than in hospitals.
- The level of professional education of staff is routinely lower in nursing homes than in hospitals.
- Frequently, there are language and cultural differences between staff and patients.
- Levels of staffing in nursing homes often are stretched to the limit.
- The nursing home industry is highly regulated and facility administrators tend to react in a highly legalistic fashion when problems and conflicts arise, for fear of sanctions, reprimands, fines, or threats of closure by state inspection/oversight teams.
- Families and friends, after initial involvement at admission, may have little or nothing to do with the day-to-day care and decisions made for nursing home residents.[5]
- Residents are not simply patients; they *live* in the facility.

An ethics committee member from a teaching facility summarized the differences between the nursing home and the teaching hospital this way: "In the hospital, the resident is the doctor; in the nursing home, the resident is the patient." If we think only of the differences between the names *nursing home* and *hospital,* a critical difference is made clear. For the patient, a hospital is expected to be temporary; a nursing home purports to be a home, at least for a time.

Ethical Issues in Chronic versus Acute Illness

The dominant characteristics of ethical concern in the acute care hospital are shaped by three factors. First, there is general agreement that the desired goal is cure or restoration of function, although there may be disagreement as to what is possible or whether the risks of treatments that have potential for obtaining either of these goals outweigh potential benefits. Rarely, however, is there disagreement as to the desirability of cure or rehabilitation for the patient or by the patient. Second, in the acute care setting there is a relatively short period of contact between hospital and patient. These increasingly shortened length of stays and the accelerated pace that are the fact of hospital life in this era of diagnosis-related groups contribute to an environment in which some issues with ethical import are not given great consideration. For example, privacy invasions, visitor restrictions, lack of clothing choices, and other limitations experienced in the hospital are less discussed (and perhaps more accepted) because they are temporary. Third, because the institutional culture of the acute care hospital is focused solely on medical treatment, medical decision making—encompassing the patient's or surrogate's right to make medical decisions as well as the health care professional's duty to pursue the patient's best interest—is the basis for almost all ethics discussion and hospital ethics committee activities.

By contrast, when the illness is chronic and the care long-term and provided outside the hospital, goals are more limited, more—and more kinds of—decisions must be made, and more people are involved in and affected by those decisions. In the case of long-term care, when neither cure nor restoration is possible, there is frequent disagreement as to what and whose goals and objectives are most important. Independence, comfort, longevity, quality of life, maintaining close relationships with family or friends, easy access to health care providers, and desires to avoid burdening the family are frequent values or goals sought by residents or their families, either separately or in combination.[6]

Whereas the acute care setting emphasizes conflicts between patient autonomy and professional beneficence, long-term health care ethics extends far beyond medical decision making. Preventing or resolving ethical conflicts in extended care settings requires knowing much more about the patient's life history and value system than may be necessary or even possible in acute care settings where the time to elicit these is simply not available. Quality-of-life issues often dominate discussion of ethics in long-term care, but so also do conflicts between and among patients, family, friends, and other caregivers, as well as choices about limited resources in the facility or the patient's family. Even the issue of placement in a nursing home may represent a conflict between what the patient wants (and is best for the patient) and what the family wants (and is best for the family). In these settings there is a broad expanse of time in which everyone's interests can be expressed and throughout which resources may be expended.

Because long-term care is to provide a home, the nursing home must be attentive to full and ongoing expression of patient/client/resident values. Providers need to be especially sensitive not only to the residents' values about a wide range of issues, but also to the interests and needs of many kinds of caregivers, including family members, which makes the usual caregiver–patient–family triangle much more complex.

Beyond this, chronic illness and long-term care present two ethical issues: the nature of dependence and the nature of capacity. These two issues have prompted a new look at the "old" principle of autonomy, defined as a spectrum along which several types of independence and dependence commingle in any given individual and in which decisional (in)capacity must repeatedly be assessed and distinguished from legal (in)competence. In long-term care, decisional capacity must be understood more richly. A recent Hastings Center research report on long-term care asserts that "nursing homes must be founded on the realization . . . that dependency has a positive and proper place in the scheme of human life."[7] This is a very different view than is usually taken in the acute care setting where dependency is to be overcome. Long-term care ethics committees will be obliged to flesh out the practical meanings of such a statement so that the wide range of decisions that are regularly made can contribute to residents' dignity, if not always conform to their preferences, and can create a broader understanding of autonomy.

Autonomy: Independence and Decisional Capacity

The principle of autonomy in chronic illness and long-term care encompasses a much wider range of ethical values and issues than is suggested by the high-profile, telescoped experience of acute care. Concerns with autonomy in the acute care setting traditionally have focused almost exclusively on medical decision making. In long-term care facilities, autonomy issues frequently focus on (personal) privacy, guardianship and alternatives to guardianship, family dynamics, balancing independence with the need to maintain a safe environment, appropriate responses over time to individuals with dementia, and disabilities that cruelly diminish a person's sense of dignity and self-control, such as incontinence, impaired memory, and unpredictable behavior.

A distinction could be made between the "biomedical ethics" of the acute care hospital and the "everyday ethics" of the long-term care facility. Yet this distinction is hard to maintain when the resident's medical care and well-being depend on long-term relationships with staff who are caregivers, friends, colleagues, and rule setters. The ethical issues of long-term care pervade all aspects of the resident's life and, because the long-term care facility is a health care setting, issues relating to medical care are likely to influence issues of daily living. For example, incontinence and dementia are both medical in origin and may be amenable to treatment, but they also have profound institutional and social implications for the resident that are not simply part of the burdens–benefits analysis. Similarly, conclusions that a patient is not able to make medical treatment decisions may lead to the assumption that the patient is unable to make decisions about daily life or even to have preferences considered. Yet patients may have some abilities to make choices even when they suffer significant impairment. Exercising even limited abilities can provide a sense of health and control. The exercise of such abilities, however, will very much be determined by others.

When autonomy issues arise, it is necessary to distinguish between *decisional autonomy* (the ability and freedom to make decisions) and *executional autonomy* (the ability to carry out and implement personal choice). Long-term care settings are generally characterized by an intense concern for ordinary quality-of-life issues: May I eat when and what I want? Must I have a designated roommate? When can I go out for a walk? Why can't I wake up and go to sleep when I want to? Why can't I wash my clothes in the bathroom sink? What can I wear to dinner? Do I have to take a bath? When can I have help in using the telephone?[8]

Autonomy in long-term care, which is the right and the capacity of an individual to direct the course of his or her life, may include, to varying degrees, both decisional autonomy and executional autonomy. Most of the examples given above involve executional autonomy. The question is whether a person is permitted (and perhaps assisted so that the permission is not hollow) to do these things. It is not whether the person has a right to choose but whether he or she is actually able to do it. The traditional view of autonomy — the right to be left alone and not be constrained by others — does the bed-bound, institutionally constrained resident little good. Autonomy for this patient is more a matter of *positive rights* (ensuring access to something) than of *negative rights* (not being interfered with).

Because acute care ethics has focused so intensely on decisional autonomy and negative rights, those in long-term care who are able to make decisions but unable to execute or implement their wishes are at great risk of having their autonomy ignored or discounted. Informed consent as a procedural guide is not sufficient in the context of chronic disability and long-term care to ensure respect for patients in the same way that it has been relied on in the acute care hospital. The protesting patient in the acute care hospital is likely to receive attention just because he or she is expected to regain executional autonomy; the protesting patient in the long-term care facility may be more likely to protest in vain. In addition, the hospitalized patient protests what is being offered, whereas the long-term care resident protests what is *not* being offered. Even in legal terms, a distinction exists: giving treatment that is refused is a battery; not giving opportunities that are desired is not (although it may be a civil rights violation).

Professional Authority and Caregiver Relationships

Physicians and nurses in long-term care have moral and legal responsibility for their patients. However, because of the structure of long-term care, they often are not available. That creates tension between them and the staff who are regularly with the patients making the hour-by-hour and day-by-day decisions. Physicians and nurses would like to control those decisions, limiting other caregivers' discretion, but they are too far away to exert such control. Although they may be willing to accept patients' wishes as the primary value, the more paternalistic or beneficent orientation of the long-term care facility and its staff may dominate. As a result, the relationships between physicians and nurses who are essentially outside the facility and the staff within it may be contentious.

Furthermore, as the presence and influence of physicians and nurses diminish, other parties will ask and expect to be heard. Although families may sometimes be intimidated by the highly educated professionals in the acute care setting with its technological orientation, they are less likely to be deferential to caregivers in the nursing home, who often do not have high levels of professional education. In addition, in home care settings where families, neighbors, and close friends function as health care providers, they begin to take on a dual status (they are both personally attached to the patient and have "professional-like" relationships with the patient). This, too, must alter our understanding of the ethics of the patient–provider relationship.

These kinds of issues will be reflected in the agendas of long-term care ethics committees in the years to come. Ethics committees and consultants will be asked to focus on treatment decisions and on the everyday ethical issues facing clients and providers. They may find themselves writing DNR policies, or they may "deliberate about who should get the next single room, how roommates are selected, and how to handle the disturbing person with Alzheimer's disease so as to respect the dignity and autonomy of all. They could consider whether a resident should be forced to get up for breakfast because the facility is required to serve the first meal of the morning no later than 14 hours after the last substantial meal of the evening, whether a nurse's aide can vary her routine to attend to a resident's request, and how the staff should balance conflicting demands of family and resident."[9] They will need to improve problem-solving methods within institutions and among multiple interested parties, perhaps by incorporating into their formal activities the skills and principles routinely employed by trained mediators in dispute resolution.[10] And they will need to incorporate the patient's voice and values, even when he or she lacks many capacities.

In long-term care, there are more decisions to make, but more time to make them. There is more time for extended formal and informal conversation and assessment of capacity, and the opportunity to wait for periods of lucidity when a patient's wishes may be ascertained and acted on. Thus, long-term care ethics committees may more regularly be of help in individual cases than are committees in the acute care hospital, where time is often too short to permit their involvement.

Nursing Home Ethics Committees

Ethics committees for nursing homes are fast becoming a reality. Growth is certain to accelerate in the next five years, and the impact of ethical issues in long-term care on the more traditional medical ethics agenda is already being felt. For example, hospitals are beginning to incorporate new definitions and procedures for determining decisional capacity, and institutions throughout the community are beginning to develop interagency transfer policies that may start with creating portable DNR orders and could culminate in calls for a common and portable medical record.

Some committees already exist within and serve a single nursing home. Because many nursing homes are owned by a corporation, the corporation may have a single ethics committee for its multistate business. Other committees reflect and serve a consortium of facilities within a given community or region. Still others are organized around state agencies responsible for setting policy for and monitoring individual institutions. For example, some state agencies on aging, which provide ombudspersons statewide, are in the early stages of developing statewide ethics committees for nursing homes. These committees, however, are not so much created to deal with individual cases as to ensure that all nursing home policies and regulations are sufficiently informed by considerations of ethics. The New Jersey statewide home care association also created such a committee.

The practical realities of nursing homes discussed above argue against structuring committees and planning activities in ways that mirror hospital ethics committees.[11] These differences must influence structural, procedural, and substantive considerations as nursing homes engage ethics consultants and/or develop ethics committees.

Membership

Few if any facilities employ their own ethics consultant, and within most facilities it is difficult to find a sufficiently broad representation of disciplines to create an adequately diverse and multidisciplinary committee membership. As a result, many committees will seek more outside community members (including residents' families) than would a hospital ethics committee to complement the limited internal resources. This infusion of community members may help counter the highly structured and hierarchical culture that is even more characteristic of nursing homes than of hospitals.

The ultimate membership of existing nursing home committees could become, through this infusion of community members, similar to that of hospital ethics committees, although there are likely to be proportionally more nurses and fewer physicians involved (rarely will such a committee be dominated by physicians). Whereas in hospital ethics committees it is sometimes difficult to secure participation from a key administrator, the nursing home administrator is almost always a leading figure on the committee. The administrator may, however, contribute to power imbalances similar to those inherent in physician-dominated committees. Because of the residential nature of such facilities and the need for ongoing decision making, and given a history of resident participation in the life of the facility, there is the strong expectation by advocacy groups, regulating agencies, and sometimes the residents and families that residents will play an important role as members of these committees. Relationships between professionals and residents and their families on these committees are (or should be) much more symmetrical and reciprocal than is the case in hospitals, and committee membership and process are bound to reflect this.

Ombudspersons

Long-term care facilities have an additional resource for their ethics committee—the Ombudsman Program, which under the Older Americans Act requires ombudspersons to investigate and resolve complaints made by or on behalf of residents. Ombudspersons, like ethics committees (especially those that see themselves as patient advocates), generally are not charged with making decisions for the residents but, rather, are responsible for representing residents' needs and wishes. Increasingly, these patient representatives are asking: "How can the ombudsmen work through ethical issues—whether the issue is one of individual case advocacy or one of broader scope like legislative, or systems, advocacy?"[12] The process recommended by Hunt for an ombudsperson performing case consultation on biomedical issues is nearly identical to that used by an ethics consultant or committee case review, and is outlined below:[13]

1. Represent the resident.
2. Collect relevant background medical information including proposed interventions, expected outcomes, and available alternatives.
3. Involve appropriate stakeholders and interested parties (such as resident, family, direct care personnel, medical personnel, clergy, or friends) in discussing the situation.
4. Involve outside resources as necessary.
5. Maintain the focus on the resident.

Most frequently, the ombudsperson finds himself or herself involved in "balancing conflicting needs, rights, and interests; deciphering best interest, or what 'good' prevails; distinguishing what's feasible from what is most desirable if the two are incompatible; and asking pertinent questions and/or rallying outside resources."[14]

Ombudspersons are being encouraged to develop legislative and systems management skills, and some groups are recommending the establishment of an ethics committee for an entire statewide Ombudsman Program, which would concentrate on education, policy and standards review, and retrospective case review.[15] Any nursing home ethics committee would do well to involve the facility ombudsperson in its program, either formally or informally. Ultimately, it may be the ombudsperson who can help small nursing homes develop interfacility ethics committees.

Issues and Areas of Concern

The functions of ethics committees in the long-term care setting are likely to be essentially the same as those in acute care hospitals: education, policy recommendations, and case review. However, they are likely to manifest somewhat differently because of the above-described differences.

Many government-mandated policies and procedures regulate nursing home activities. Some of these, such as the Patient Self-Determination Act, could be of special use to an ethics committee. For example, there is an elaborate and highly regulated admissions process which, given constraints of time and staff, is often rushed and unduly coercive.[16] A nursing home ethics committee could be helpful in reviewing the contents of such an admissions contract and finding ways to execute it more meaningfully. This could be the locus for explaining initial and subsequent determination of decisional (in)capacity; appointment and use of surrogate decision makers; the facility's conformity with federal and state Patients' Bill of Rights and informed consent procedures; patient-executed advance directives; and the required involvement of the resident and/or family in the development of a long-term care plan.

These are such central ethical issues that a committee might well spend many months simply trying to ensure that those who enter the nursing home genuinely understand what this admission means to them with regard to decision making solely at the medical level. It may be that a nursing home ethics committee may initially be most effective in providing education and developing policies that will ensure education of residents and staff on the current areas of ethical consensus and legal regulation.

Several substantive areas of medical ethics loom large in long-term care settings. These include determining and documenting decisional incapacity; determining surrogates for residents who lack decision-making capacity and have no family or friends to act as surrogate; and developing transportable medical records and treatment orders (especially advance directives and life-support treatment orders). Ethics committees in both acute and long-term care facilities can be expected to become more involved in these issues and to cooperate more fully in the exchange of policies and procedures.

It would be helpful to both groups if there were some interchange of members. The Orange County (California) Bioethics Network, whose original members all came from hospital ethics committees, found that resolving important ethical issues (particularly involving transfer of patients between nursing home and hospital) required inviting nursing home staff to discuss their common problems. The result was the formation of a subcommittee of the Network that solely addresses nursing home ethical issues and a steering committee for the Network that includes individuals from both groups. The Network's quarterly educational programs address issues important to both kinds of institutions.

Decision-Making Capacity

Because so many long-term care residents have impaired capacity to make decisions, it is vital that this issue be addressed. At present, there are few if any formal or uniform standards and policies for determining decisional incapacity in either acute or long-term care settings, although policies in each are beginning to pay at least lip service to the importance of determining and respecting a patient/client's decisional capacity. Nor are there standards of practice for monitoring changes in patient/client status, documenting such status, or seeing that patient/client autonomy is respected and enhanced over time as much as possible.

Long-term care facilities are just beginning to do research and staff training on this issue, and we would expect benefits to accrue to acute care facilities where assessment time is limited but the patient's right to make medical decisions is of prime concern to ethics committees. A nursing home ethics committee could be of real help in promoting such research, policy development, and training activities, and in helping those in the acute care hospital to understand how these assessments of capacity are carried out in the nursing home. (However, given that few ethics committees have much familiarity with research ethics, committees should be cautious about promoting research. As desirable as research may be, it may easily place the committee in a position of conflicting interests via the residents.)

Surrogate Decision Makers

One issue that seems more urgent in acute care facilities (where authorized informed consent is a high-profile requirement) is actually more serious in terms of sheer numbers in long-term care facilities—the problem of patients/residents who have no authorized or identified decision maker and who can no longer make decisions for themselves. Although there are no reliable figures, some analysts have estimated that between 40 and 50 percent of the country's entire institutionalized long-term care population falls into this category. When these people require medical treatment, the prospect of having to secure a court-appointed guardian in each case is a nightmare.

Ethics committees and consultants can be useful in developing and implementing policies that prevent such a situation by encouraging patient/resident-appointed surrogates; working with local and regional professionals and agencies to develop alternatives to guardianship wherever possible;[17] and reviewing and assisting the development of state "family consent" statutes that obviate the need for regular recourse to the courts and court-appointed guardians.

Guidelines for Transporting Medical Records and Honoring Patient Wishes

One area in which long-term care consortia have taken the lead in their communities is in the development of uniform guidelines for transporting medical records and honoring patient wishes whether at home, in a nursing home, in an ambulance, or in a hospital. In Sonoma County, California, between 1987 and 1989, skilled nursing facilities and acute care hospitals worked with paramedics and emergency treatment agencies to institute joint policies, procedures, and forms relating to transfers between facilities and to joint education programs.[18] Similarly, in Orange County, California, the Bioethics Network helped the county emergency medicine agency develop a program that permitted DNR orders to be honored by paramedics. This was done initially for patients in hospice or under home health care, with a planned subsequent phase-in for nursing home patients.

It may be the case that compliance with the Patient Self-Determination Act will serve to promote more universal cooperation and exchange in these areas, but the need for ethics committees and consultants to focus on patient rights as distinct from institutional expediency will remain crucial. Nursing homes may have more difficulty in freeing staff to participate in these activities than hospitals. As a result, the chairpersons of such committees will need to cast their nets widely to find additional resources. Hospital ethics committees can help their colleagues in extended care by offering to share their own expertise, inviting nursing home staff to hospital ethics committee meetings and educational programs, and inviting nursing home ethics committees to join in regional networks.

Adoption of Corporatewide Policies

A concern that seems to be relatively specific to nursing homes (especially nursing home chains) is the practice of adopting and enforcing corporatewide policies with respect to life-support treatment, regardless of the laws and practices of the states and communities in which individual facilities are located. An increasingly common strategy is to establish informal or formal ethics committees at the local level to communicate to "headquarters" what is locally required and expected with respect to advance directives and life-support treatment decisions. When this is accomplished, it is not unusual for the corporation itself to establish an ethics committee or advisory panel, composed of corporate and local facility representatives, to review policies and determine where corporatewide policies are required or where individual facilities may or should develop their own.

Such centralized committees may be helpful in ensuring consistent policies, but they also may leave the individual facilities feeling that they have little or no voice in policy making. In addition, corporate nursing home ethics committees may not act in accordance with the needs of the individual facility. For example, the specific nursing home committee may conclude that its facility needs a policy on a specific issue, whereas the central committee, which has taken the policy-making function unto itself, does not feel a similar need. The Patient Self-Determination Act should help nursing homes develop and implement policies that are appropriate to their own state laws, but nursing home chains need to find ways to promote a sense of ownership at the local level. Ethics imposed from the top is poorly understood (and usually poorly acted on).

Education

The education function of the committee may be met in many ways. Acute care hospitals often have initiated their work with bioethics study groups whose sole function is to become more familiar with the literature in the field. More recently, ethics committees have been initiated with specific tasks (for example, writing DNR policies), and self-education has been more indirect as the committee members learn from one another through the execution of the task. A New York nursing home reported on its regularly held "ethics rounds," during which specific cases were discussed with the residents of the home and their family, as well as with staff.[19] The authors describe this as an alternative to an ethics committee, but it could equally be the primary educational forum of the ethics committee. Including patients and families as participants in the discussion (rather than as the objects of the discussion) effectively demonstrates an understanding of the different role that residents occupy in the nursing home, as opposed to the hospital. However, privacy concerns would need careful attention if ongoing cases were to be used as the basis of the case conference.

If outside expertise is needed to provide education, it may be most effective to have several nursing homes join together to educate selected staff members who can then bring information back to their respective facilities. In addition, joint education sessions help nursing home staff feel less isolated with their ethical problems and provide opportunities for networking and problem solving from a broader perspective.

Transplanting the idea of ethics committees from acute care to long-term care facilities is surely justified, but the fate of this transplant is unclear because of the many differences between the two kinds of institutions. It will be some time before anyone can say with any confidence that policy writing or case review are or should be primary functions of these committees. However, education of the committee and of the staff, residents, and family on the complexity of the issues and on legal standards and ethical consensus (where it exists) is clearly an appropriate and needed function.

Research on ethics committees in acute care hospitals has been slow to develop; such research in the long-term care facility may be even slower in coming. Thus, innovation (as well as a feeling of isolation) at the facility level probably will be the norm for some time to come. Joining together with other long-term care ethics committees for education sessions or networking, working with other institutions in the geographic area to solve interfacility problems (such as the DNR order between hospital and home or nursing home), and joining or helping create local ethics committee networks that include both long-term care facilities and acute care hospitals may be the best way in the foreseeable future to reduce the sense of isolation that these committees may feel and to share the experience that each facility has gained in addressing its own ethical concerns.

Ethical Issues in Home Care

Much of what has been said above about the centrality of chronic care issues applies as well to ethics in home care, although it is somewhat less applicable to home hospice programs. Unlike the case in nursing homes, however, overcoming institutional hierarchy is not an ethics committee issue in home care because care is delivered outside the institution. Peculiar to home care are the location of service delivery (the patient's home); the caregiver mix, which includes both family and formal caregivers; and the unique ". . . interaction between the exercise of autonomy and reimbursement, regulation, environment, and technology in the home-care setting."[20]

As is the case in long-term care generally, helping the patient/client articulate his or her underlying values, preferences, and beliefs becomes more important as the time available to do so expands and as the scope of decisions affecting the person broadens. Ethics committees and consultants in both nursing homes and home care agencies are working to develop and implement various "values baseline assessment" tools.[21] Such tools include, but are not limited to, the Values History Form developed by the University of New Mexico (a copy of this form is presented in appendix 11-1 at the end of the chapter). At the University of Minnesota, Rosalie Kane is working on assessment forms that are short enough and easy enough to be used in a variety of situations. Such values assessment tools, when available, also will help sensitize staff in acute care facilities to the importance of focusing not only on specific treatment choices that patients make but also on the reasons for these choices.

Patient Assertiveness

Specific to the home care setting (and quite unlike hospitals and nursing homes) is the increased assertiveness (some would say aggressiveness) of patients who "are on their own turf and are secure in their authority. They are likely to hold firm and resist the judgments of their professional caregivers if these are at odds with their own wishes. If home health care personnel override the patients' wishes, especially in their own homes, this act may be regarded as highly assaultive."[22] Thus patient advocacy in home care is different from advocacy in a hospital or nursing home.

In the home care setting, there is the additional need for a community ethic that balances the rights of vulnerable and frail citizens to remain independent and free from institutionalization, with the duties of caregivers to respond to cases of abuse and neglect. Conflicts with regard to when a person must give up living at home in order to live a safer, healthier, or more dignified life (at least from some perspective) are increasingly common as the very old outlive family members and friends and thus have no one to provide them with the vital link that would make it possible for them to stay in their homes. A real service provided by an ethics committee serving home care clients and providers would be to help the community at large develop a "community ethic to guide community-based healthcare so that it preserves dignity, fosters humane standards of care, and respects the individual's right to autonomy"[23] in such circumstances.

Role of Family and Friends

Further distinguishing home care is the role of family and friends as primary caregivers. Whereas in hospitals and nursing homes professional caregivers provide most of the care, at home the family must bear much of the responsibility for ongoing care. Potential for abuse increases with such stress, and professional health care providers must be able to balance their own rights as caregivers with those of the family and the patient. In addition, when family members become caregivers, routine views of patients' privacy concerns may be sharply altered for the caregivers, but not for the patients.

In the acute care and nursing home setting, family members are often privy to information only with the consent of the patient, whereas professional caregivers must have access to the information to provide care. But having family members share the role of caregiver eliminates this distinction, at least at the theoretical level. One privacy issue that arose early in the AIDS epidemic was whether family members who were providing home care had the right to know about the patient's diagnosis if the patient was unwilling to share that information. An early consensus appeared to be that the family member *as caregiver* was entitled to the information (because the caregiver was at risk of infection), but that the family member *as relative* was not entitled to the information. However, this is less clear these days with the current understanding that universal infection control procedures are appropriate for all, including those being cared for at home by family members and that, at least in theory, such procedures obviate the need for caregivers to have specific information on HIV status. However, the person who cares for one family member is differently situated than the person who cares for many strangers.

It should be emphasized, however, that in home care the truly interactive and reciprocal nature of care giving stands out more than in any other setting. Any ethics committee or consultant must understand this, and should consider including (either on the committee or as an available resource) community members and support agencies that have direct experience with these issues. As the site of health care delivery moves away from institutions, the need for community and lay representation increases.

Additional Issues

Any ethics committee or advisor to home health care agencies must have a real appreciation for the intricacies and failures of distributive justice in the current health care delivery system:

"Nowhere in the health system is there a greater gap between the needs of the patient and the available resources than in long-term home healthcare."[24] Added to these difficulties is the increasing regulation of the industry since its formalization with the passage of Medicare and Medicaid in 1965, as well as the constant worker shortages.

Although residents of nursing homes may suffer environmental and institutional constraints on their autonomy, there still is the likelihood that ongoing relationships with the staff will be formed and that a rich profile and understanding of residents' values can be developed. In home health care, regulations, compounded by funding and worker shortages, make home health care agencies extremely productivity conscious. Nurses often have a quota of visits to make in a week and are likely to be very task/time oriented.

Precisely those activities so important in the management of chronic illness (maintaining patient autonomy, determining and monitoring decisional capacity, and educating and becoming acquainted with the patient and his or her family) are prohibitively time-consuming activities and often are not billable. Moreover, the patient population in home health care is routinely more acutely ill and dependent on increasingly high levels of technology (ventilators, feeding pumps, intravenous fluids) delivered in an environment (the home) that is not structured for this type of care. Thus, the professionals' abilities to develop and sustain relationships with patients and their families are even further strained, because the time available to professionals may be disproportionately needed for technological issues.

An additional issue for home health agency ethics committees may relate to concerns of the staff about their own professional obligations with respect to clients' understanding of services. For example, individuals who enter hospice programs under Medicare reimbursement must relinquish access to acute care "curative" treatment for a period of time and may be required to agree to DNR orders. How thoroughly clients understand the nature of the decision they are making is somewhat problematic, insofar as real understanding takes place over a period of time. But clients often sign the admission agreements at the beginning of that period of time, not at the end, because the discussion can continue only after entry into the program. Family members, not the individual patient, may be the ones who really understand the nature of the decision that has been made and this may be problematic for professionals.

Other even more complex concerns of home health care professionals can involve agencies' offering services that are only marginally available. For example, clients may be told that they have 24-hour-a-day access to nurses, whereas nurses may be unwilling to make night home calls in areas that are at least perceived to be dangerous after dark. Respecting both clients' needs for services and professionals' needs for safety can be very difficult and, as safety concerns in the AIDS epidemic have shown, those who are not at risk often are the most assertive about the need to rise to "professional standards."

Home health care should teach us even more about how to conceptualize and understand ethical issues in the context of relationships. This idea contrasts with the more prevalent view in bioethics that ethics is about "rights bearers" whose relationships to others have no effect on ethical constructs, as if all people were strangers, isolated from one another and without value-related bonds.

Community Ethics Committees

Several groups around the country have been experimenting with community-based ethics committees. One of these, the Arizona Health Decisions (AHD) project, has been in existence since 1986. In some sense, such committees respond directly to the need for a social ethics context—to provide a resource that comes from and serves the community at large and to help the community discuss and develop an appropriate community health care ethic.

The AHD announced that its goal was to return to the community both the responsibility and the authority for decision making in matters of personal and public health. Over the past several years, the AHD has undertaken public bioethics education and has established and trained a community volunteer bioethics committee. Community and committee education has included sessions on theoretical ethics, applied decision making, review of relevant case law, religious doctrines, communication skill building, values clarification, overview of professional systems, overview of family systems, loss/dying/grief education, resource allocation in health care, and mediation skills in case consultation.

Such groups or committees can be useful in a number of areas, especially as more issues reach the public policy arena (for example, voluntary active euthanasia initiatives such as those that have been placed on the ballot in Washington State and in California). These committees can provide communitywide education on a scale not possible for institutional ethics committees, whose time and energy are already stretched. They can develop materials that address a broad spectrum of interest and needs, not necessarily driven by narrower institutional issues; they can provide speakers' bureaus that include a wide representation of community health care professionals; they can serve as a community-based advocacy group that can lobby and be seen as broadly representative of all citizens, independent of single-interest groups; and they can offer education and consultation services to institutions (especially long-term and home care) that are considering or beginning to establish internal or cooperative ethics committees. Although such community-based ethics committees are the newest and therefore most untested groups, their noninstitutional, grass-roots origins and nature make them the most interesting to track over the next few years.

Conclusion

There is no question that the issues, locations, and interested parties in long-term care delivery will only increase in number and diversity in the years to come. It is difficult to predict exactly how ethics committees will function in such a different environment. It is apparent in the acute care hospital that an effective ethics committee depends on several members having a very strong commitment to realizing ethical concerns in their workplace. Whether nursing home committees will be able to find such individuals within their ranks is questionable, given the enormous demands on their time. Finding them from outside the facilities may be a solution for keeping the committees active and informed, but it will be difficult if the most strongly committed individuals are not themselves working within the facility. Creating multifacility committees may be a better way to achieve both strength and longevity for many institutions.

Despite this uncertainty about how the committees will function over time, the advice given in years past to fledgling (hospital) ethics committees is equally appropriate for nursing home ethics committees: learn about yourselves and your values first, and always attend carefully to the genuine and individual needs and interests of the involved parties. Let these needs and interests dictate the committee's form and the facility's policies and procedures.

The community's perception of its most important problems is the first issue to address. If nursing home residents and staff believe that, for example, roommate selection is their most pressing issue with respect to resident dignity, that is the issue to address, even if administrators would prefer policy development around the requirements of the Patient Self-Determination Act. The internal community—whether nursing home, home health care program, or community—must set the initial agenda so that the community owns its ethical standards. The alternative—and one that has already been seen in acute care hospitals—is a committee created to respond to tasks and standards imposed solely through legal needs or regulatory or bureaucratic requirements. This results in an ethics committee that is not taken seriously by either its members or its institution.

Exercises

1. Recent research has shown that restraints are used much more extensively in U.S. nursing homes than in similar facilities in other Western countries. Some research suggests that residents placed in restraints may in fact be at increased risk of harm as a result of the restraints. Regulations discouraging or prohibiting use of mechanical or chemical restraints

on an "as needed" basis are increasingly being issued by regulatory agencies. Justifications for mechanical restraints are usually based on preventing harm to the client/resident.

As an exercise in refocusing the problem, committee members can take several actual cases of patients with whom restraints are being used and brainstorm to explore other ways in which risk of harm to the patient could be reduced. The object of such an exercise is to expand the range of possible methods through which the legitimate desire to protect could be realized without essentially imprisoning the resident.

2. A social worker in a home health hospice agency comes to the ethics committee with a report that one of her clients has talked to her about the desirability of suicide and the need to obtain adequate drugs for a fatal overdose. The patient has a terminal illness and has refused further treatment. From her conversation with the nurse on the case, the social worker learns that the client has complained to the nurse that her pain medication is inadequate. Together, the social worker and nurse surmise that the client may be holding back on taking the pain medication in order to accumulate enough of the drug to commit suicide. The social worker is not willing to assist the client in committing suicide, nor does she think the nurse should, but she contends that if that is what the client wants to do, they should not interfere with her. The nurse, on the other hand, believes that allowing a patient to commit suicide by not acting is antithetical to the hospice ethical standards and to her own professional obligations. How should they resolve this conflict? Would it help if the agency had a policy dealing with patients' suicidal desires? What should the policy attempt to achieve?

3. Committee members should make a list of what they think are the three or four most important ethical issues to staff, residents, residents' families, and administrators. When they have completed these lists, make a master list for each group. Is there any consensus on what issues are important for each group? Are there issues that are important to all four groups? If the committee conducted a survey of each group, would the groups agree on what issues were important to them? For example, how well do staff know what the most pressing ethical concerns are for administrators or families? Do administrators know what staffs' concerns are? How can lists or questionnaires help improve communication on what is important to different people?

Notes and References

1. American Association of Retired Persons. *Highlights,* May–June 1991, p. 10.

2. American Association of Retired Persons, p. 2.

3. Cotler, M. When policies don't work out: finding the source of the problem. *Ethical Currents* 26:1–2, Spring 1991.

4. Pember, C. H., III, and Fonner, E., Jr. Prevailing issues in long-term care. *Health Progress* June 1992, pp. 38–42. In a survey of CEOs of long-term care facilities, ethical issues involving forgoing treatment was the number 5 issue; the other nine issues were essentially all about finances, either directly or indirectly.

5. Meece, K. Long-term care bioethics: a cooperative model. *Ethical Currents* 20:1, Fall 1989.

6. Meece, pp. 4–5.

7. Collopy, B., Boyle, P., and Jennings, B. New directions in nursing home ethics: special supplement. *Hastings Center Report* (suppl.), Mar.–Apr., pp. 1–15.

8. Kane, R. A., and Caplan, A. L. Ethical issues arising in the daily lives of nursing home residents. In: *Everyday Ethics: Resolving Dilemmas in Nursing Home Life.* New York City: Springer Publishing Co., 1990, p. 38.

9. Kane, R. A., Freeman, I. C., Caplan, A. L., Aroskot, M. A., and Urv-Wong, E. R. Everyday autonomy in nursing homes. *Generations* (suppl.), 1990, p. 71.

10. West, M. B., and Gibson, J. M. Facilitating medical ethics case review: what ethics committees can learn from mediation and facilitation techniques. *Cambridge Quarterly* 1(1):63–74, 1992.

11. For a discussion of membership and other organizational issues, see *Ethics Committees: Allies in Long-Term Care: A Guidebook to Forming an Ethics Committee*. This booklet was published in 1990 by the AARP and the American Association of Homes for the Aging. An inexpensive companion video also is available from AARP.

12. Hunt, S. S. Working through ethical dilemmas in ombudsperson practice. Prepared for the National Center for Long Term Care Ombudsperson Resources, 1989, p. 22.

13. Hunt, p. 32.

14. Hunt, p. 32.

15. For a full proposal for a statewide ombudsperson ethics committee, see Hunt, pp. 37–40.

16. Ambrogi, D. M. Nursing home admissions: problematic process and agreements. *Generations* (suppl.), 1990, pp. 72–74.

17. Medical treatment guardian projects have been developed in New Mexico and Minnesota and are currently under study in other states.

18. Meece, p. 1.

19. Libow, L. S., Olson, E., and Neufeld, R. R., Marnco-Greenfield, T., Meyers, H., Gordon, N., and Barnett, P. Ethics rounds at the nursing home: an alternative to an ethics committee. *Journal of American Geriatrics Society* 40(1):95–97, 1992.

20. Young, P. A. Home-care characteristics that shape the exercise of autonomy. *Generations* (suppl.), 1990, p. 17.

21. The Values History Form (in appendix 11-1) developed at the University of New Mexico's Institute of Public Law and the work being done by Rosalie Kane at the University of Minnesota are examples of such tools and processes. Also, see: Palaez, M., and David, D. *Facilitator's Guide: Identifying Clients' Values and Preferences*. San Jose, CA: Southeast Florida Center on Aging and the Gerontology Education and Training Center, 1991.

22. Young, p. 18.

23. Young, p. 18.

24. Young, p. 20.

Appendix 11-1. Values History Form

Name: _____

Date: _____

If someone assisted you in completing this form, please fill in his or her name, address, and relationship to you.

Name: _____

Address: _____

Relationship: _____

The purpose of this form is to assist you in thinking about and writing down what is important to you about your health. If you should at some time become unable to make health care decisions for yourself, your thoughts as expressed on this form may help others make a decision for you in accordance with what you would have chosen.

The first section of this form asks whether you have already expressed your wishes concerning medical treatment through either written or oral communications and, if not, whether you would like to do so now. The second section of this form provides an opportunity for you to discuss your values, wishes, and preferences in a number of different areas such as your personal relationships, your overall attitude toward life, and your thoughts about illness.

Suggestions for Use

The Values History Form was developed at the Center for Health Law and Ethics, University of New Mexico School of Law and Ethics, University of New Mexico School of Law. The form is *not a legal document*, although it may be used to supplement a living will or a durable power of attorney for health care, if you have these. Also, the Values History Form is not copyrighted, and you are encouraged to make additional copies for friends and relatives to use.

Why a Values History Form?
The Values History Form recognizes that medical decisions we make for ourselves are based on those beliefs, preferences, and values that matter most to us: How do we feel about independence and control? About pain, illness, dying, and death? What in life gives us pleasure? Sorrow? A discussion of these and other values can provide important information for those who might, in the future, have to make medical decisions for us when we are no longer able to do so.

Further, a discussion of the questions asked on the Values History Form can provide a solid basis for families, friends, physicians, and others when making such medical decisions. By talking about such issues ahead of time, family disagreements may be minimized. And when such decisions do need to be made, the burden of responsibility may be lessened because others feel confident of your wishes.

How Do I Fill Out the Values History Form?
Section 1 allows you to record both written and oral instructions you might already have prepared. Simply answer the questions. If you have not yet written or talked about these issues, you might wait to complete this section at a later date, perhaps after you have completed Section 2.

Section 2 asks a number of questions about issues such as: Your attitude toward your health; your feelings about your health care providers; your thoughts about independence and control; personal relationships; your overall attitude toward life; your attitude toward illness/dying/death; your religious background and beliefs; your living environment; your attitude toward finances; your wishes concerning your funeral.

There are a number of ways in which you might begin to answer these questions. Perhaps you would like to write out some of your own thoughts before you talk with anyone else. Or you might ask family and friends to come together and talk about your—and their—responses to the questions.

Often simply making copies of the Values History Form available to others is enough to get people talking about a subject that, for many of us, is difficult and painful to consider. The most important thing to remember is that it is easier to talk about these issues *before* a medical crisis occurs. Feel free to add questions and comments of your own to those already provided.

What Should I Do with My Completed Values History Form?
Make certain that all those who might be involved in future medical decisions made on your behalf are aware of your wishes: family, friends, physicians and other health care providers, your lawyer, your

pastor. If appropriate, provide written copies to these people. But remember that each of us continues to grow and change, and so the Values History Form should be discussed and updated fairly regularly, as preferences and values evolve. Consider attaching a copy of it to your living will or durable power of attorney for health care, if you have one, or filing the Values History Form with your important medical papers.

What If I Do Not Have a Living Will or Durable Power of Attorney for Health Care?
Whether you sign either of these is entirely up to you, and laws governing these vary from state to state. For information and assistance, the following agencies might be of help:

Choice in Dying
250 West 57th Street, New York City, NY 10107
(212/366-5540)

This agency will provide legal information about living wills and durable powers of attorney for health care, as applicable in your own state. Please write to them at the above address. Because of the recent large volume of requests, expect a 4- to 6-week turnaround time. If you have an emergency, you may telephone them, but they caution that it is very difficult to get through on the telephone.

American Association of Retired Persons
1909 K Street, N.W., Washington, DC 20049

For a single, free copy of the health care power of attorney booklet, please send a postcard with your name and address to AARP Fulfillment (stock no. D13895). You might also contact your local office of senior affairs, your state or area agency on aging, agencies providing legal services for the elderly, or your personal attorney.

Who Should Consider Preparing a Values History Form?
Everyone. While it has been customary to focus on older people, it is just as important that younger people discuss these issues and make their wishes known. Often some of the most difficult medical decisions must be made on behalf of these younger patients. If they had talked with families and friends, these decision makers could feel reassured they were following the patient's wishes.

We hope this Values History Form is of help to you, your families, and friends. Many people have commented that it is important to reflect not so much on "How I want to die," but rather on "How I want to *live* until I die."

Section 1

A. Written Legal Documents
   Have you written any of the following legal documents?

   _____

   If so, please complete the requested information.

   Living Will
   Date written: _____
   Document location: _____
   Comments: (for example, any limitations, special requests, etc.)

   _____

   _____

   Durable Power of Attorney
   Date written: _____
   Document location: _____
   Comments: (for example, whom have you named to be your decision maker?)

   _____

   _____

Durable Power of Attorney for Health Care Decisions
Date written: _____
Document location: _____
Comments: (for example, whom have you named to be your decision maker?)
_____
_____

Organ Donations
Date written: _____
Document location: _____
Comments: (for example, any limitations on which organs you would like to donate)
_____
_____

B. Wishes Concerning Specific Medical Procedures

If you have ever expressed your wishes, either in writing or orally, concerning any of the following medical procedures, please complete the requested information. If you have not previously indicated your wishes on these procedures and would like to do so now, please complete this information.

Organ Donation
To whom expressed: _____
If oral, when? _____
If written, when? _____
Documentation location: _____
Comments: _____
_____

Kidney Dialysis
To whom expressed: _____
If oral, when? _____
If written, when? _____
Documentation location: _____
Comments: _____
_____

Cardiopulmonary Resuscitation (CPR)
To whom expressed: _____
If oral, when? _____
If written, when? _____
Documentation location: _____
Comments: _____
_____

Respirators
To whom expressed: _____
If oral, when? _____
If written, when? _____
Documentation location: _____
Comments: _____
_____

Artificial Nutrition
To whom expressed: _____
If oral, when? _____
If written, when? _____
Documentation location: _____
Comments: _____
_____

Artificial Hydration

To whom expressed: _____

If oral, when? _____

If written, when? _____

Documentation location: _____

Comments: _____

_____

C. General Comments

Do you wish to make any general comments about the information you provided in this section?

_____

_____

_____

Section 2

A. Your Overall Attitude toward Your Health

1. How would you describe your current health status? If you currently have any medical problems, how would you describe them?

_____

_____

2. If you have current medical problems, in what ways, if any, do they affect your ability to function?

_____

_____

3. How do you feel about your current health status?

_____

_____

4. How well are you able to meet the basic necessities of life—eating, food preparation, sleeping, personal hygiene, and so forth?

_____

_____

5. Do you wish to make any general comments about your overall health?

_____

_____

B. Your Perception of the Role of Your Doctor and Other Health Caregivers

1. Do you like your doctors? _____

_____

2. Do you trust your doctors? _____

_____

3. Do you think your doctors should make the final decision concerning any treatment you might need? _____

_____

4. How do you relate to your caregivers, including nurses, therapists, chaplains, social workers, etc.?

_____

_____

5. Do you wish to make any general comments about your doctor and other health caregivers?

_____

_____

C. Your Thoughts about Independence and Control

1. How important is independence and self-sufficiency in your life? _____
_____

2. If you were to experience decreased physical and mental abilities, how would that affect your attitude toward independence and self-sufficiency? _____
_____

3. Do you wish to make any general comments about the value of independence and control in your life? _____
_____

D. Your Personal Relationships

1. Do you expect that your friends, family, and/or others will support your decisions regarding medical treatment you may need now or in the future? _____
_____

2. Have you made any arrangements for your family or friends to make medical treatment decisions on your behalf? If so, who has agreed to make decisions for you and in what circumstances?
_____
_____

3. What, if any, unfinished business from the past are you concerned about (for example, personal and family relationships, business and legal matters)? _____
_____

4. What role do your friends and family play in your life? _____
_____

5. Do you wish to make any general comments about the personal relationships in your life?
_____
_____

E. Your Overall Attitude toward Life

1. What activities do you enjoy (for example, hobbies, watching television, and so on)?
_____
_____

2. Are you happy to be alive? _____
_____

3. Do you feel that life is worth living? _____
_____

4. How satisfied are you with what you have achieved in your life? _____
_____

5. What makes you laugh or cry? _____
_____

6. What do you fear most? What frightens or upsets you? _____
_____

7. What goals do you have for the future? _____
_____

8. Do you wish to make any general comments about your attitude toward life? _____
_____

F. Your Attitude toward Illness, Dying, and Death

1. What will be important to you when you are dying (for example, physical comfort, no pain, family members present, and so on)? _____

    _____

2. Where would you prefer to die? _____

    _____

3. What is your attitude toward death? _____

    _____

4. How do you feel about the use of life-sustaining measures in the face of:
    Terminal illness? _____
    Permanent coma? _____
    Irreversible chronic illness (for example, Alzheimer's disease)? _____

5. Do you wish to make any general comments about your attitude toward illness, dying, and death?

    _____

    _____

G. Your Religious Background and Beliefs

1. What is your religious background? _____

    _____

2. How do your religious beliefs affect your attitude toward serious or terminal illness?

    _____

    _____

3. Does your attitude toward death find support in your religion? _____

    _____

4. How does your faith community, church, or synagogue view the role of prayer or religious sacraments in an illness? _____

    _____

5. Do you wish to make any general comments about your religious background and beliefs?

    _____

    _____

H. Your Living Environment

1. What has been your living situation over the past 10 years (for example, lived alone, lived with others, and so forth)? _____

    _____

2. How difficult is it for you to maintain the kind of environment for yourself that you find comfortable? Does any illness or medical problem you have now mean that it will be harder in the future?

    _____

    _____

3. Do you wish to make any general comments about your living environment? _____

    _____

I. Your Attitude concerning Finances

1. How much do you worry about having enough money to provide for your care? _____

    _____

2. Would you prefer to spend less money on your care so that more money can be saved for the benefit of your relatives and/or friends? _____
_____

3. Do you wish to make any general comments concerning your finances and the cost of health care?
_____
_____

J. Your Wishes concerning Your Funeral

1. What are your wishes concerning your funeral and burial or cremation? _____
_____

2. Have you made your funeral arrangements? If so, with whom? _____
_____

3. Do you wish to make any general comments about how you would like your funeral and burial or cremation to be arranged or conducted? _____
_____

Optional Questions

1. How would you like your obituary (announcement of your death) to read? _____
_____

2. Write yourself a brief eulogy (a statement about yourself to be read at your funeral).
_____
_____

Suggestions for Use

After you have completed this form, you may wish to provide copies to your doctors and other health caregivers, your family, your friends, and your attorney. If you have a living will or durable power of attorney for health care decisions, you may wish to attach a copy of this form to those documents.

_____

Source: Adapted from the University of New Mexico School of Law, Albuquerque, New Mexico.

12

The Future of Ethics Committees: The Next Generation

Are ethics committees a permanent fixture in health care? Historian David Rothman, in *Strangers at the Bedside,* claims that ethics committees are a central societal response to the legal and ethical quandaries inherent in advanced medical technology and in the U.S. health care system.[1] Dismay with physicians and the health care system generally has led to widespread fears that patient care decisions will be made by physicians who are strangers to the patients and their family and whose values are foreign to them. Or, even worse, those decisions will be made by anonymous individuals in a government or corporate office that is indifferent to the personal values and well-being of patients but infinitely concerned about a financial bottom line and saving money. Ethics committees appear to be a way of protecting patients from this type of disrespect. Suggestions and proposals for mandating ethics committees are common.[2] An early version of the federal Patient Self-Determination Act even mandated ethics committee formation. Thus, ethics committees would appear to be a phenomenon with a secure future.

Uncertainties about Role

In the midst of all this ethics committee support, however, we should be cautious. Although there is general agreement on what ethics committees should do, there are very little empirical data on what ethics committees actually do and, more important, virtually no data—either empiric or anecdotal—on how and why they do it. Furthermore, there is great disagreement in the literature as to how ethics committees should do what they do. Leaders in bioethics as well as ethics committee members themselves have very different understandings of what an ethics committee is about: its mission, its ethos, and its metaphor. It is very probable that most people in this field have an idea or understanding of the concept *ethics committee* that is coterminous with the actual ethics committee of which they are a member or (for those who are not members of such committees) with an ethics committee of which they have imagined being a member. Some think of committees as bureaucratic bodies; some think of them as small groups with considerable intimacy; some think of them as groups of ethics experts; some think of them as hospital peacemakers; and some think of them as minicourts.

Furthermore, ethics committees have many critics. Fears about what ethics committees do or might do often arise from these diverse understandings and often are rooted in nothing more than fancy. For example, at a conference in 1992, a prominent bioethicist speaking on historical features of bioethics noted that health care ethics committees were a unique contribution of bioethics, albeit a bad one. He was certainly free to have such an opinion, but there was no evidence that he had any experience with actual committees on which to base his opinion. Rather, it was his *idea* of an ethics committee that worried him.

The multidisciplinarity that is understood to be an essential quality of ethics committees may in fact be the source of much of this uncertainty. Physicians and nurses see ethics committees through their professional eyes as forums for the exercise of technical expertise. Lawyers see them through their professional eyes as assemblies for legal review and legislation. And philosophers and clergy (for the most part teachers) see them through their professional eyes as classrooms for adult learning. Furthermore, these three primary models for understanding ethics committees are matched to the committees' primary functions: education (the educator's view), policy making (the lawyer's view), and consultation (the clinical expert's view).[3]

What is important is that all these various perceptions are in the minds of the observers. There is no agreed-on pattern or blueprint explaining how to form a recognizable ethics committee. Ethics committees began with a name, three activities, and a fairly well-articulated description of an important problem related to health care decision making—forgoing life-sustaining treatment. The name *ethics committee* does not explain how this phenomenon is to go about its work. Indeed, the name may get in the way; it connotes a kind of bureaucratic conventionality and implies that resolving ethical dilemmas is the essence of its activities. Perhaps the name is inappropriate, because these functions can be achieved in many different ways and informed by very different values. The articulated problem can be addressed by all three functions, but also by other groups in the hospital as well as in society. Knowing how ethics committees began does not ultimately help us know what they should be doing, how they should be doing it, or where they should go from here.

Concerns and Critics

It is clear that the critics do not object to ethics committees' providing education, for themselves or others, although they do object to it not being done well enough. Education, like mom and apple pie, is always seen as a good thing. Nobody else appears to want to be charged with providing it, so education probably is safely within the orbit of the ethics committee.

Policy or guideline writing is not particularly controversial either, at least at this time. However, as ethics committees begin to write policies on issues beyond the forgoing life-sustaining treatment cluster, that is, on issues where there is no general consensus on the appropriate thrust of the policy or the criteria that underlie it, problems could arise. For example, if ethics committees were to recommend policies requiring that health care professionals be tested for HIV or hepatitis B in the absence of specific legislation requiring or prohibiting it, committees might begin to hear that some people think that they are overreaching their charge. Similarly, if committees were to address at the policy level questions of futile treatment beyond the physiologically futile attempt to provide CPR, commentators might find policy and guideline writing a less desirable ethics committee activity. The general approval for committees' writing policies and guidelines is largely based on the belief that there is an existing ethical standard they will follow. Bioethics theorists may trust ethics committees to create only those policies that give voice to what is already accepted as ethical in the field of bioethics. If the committees are to do their own thinking about what is ethical, this function may become much more contentious.

But there are current criticisms and worries as well. Bioethics theorists such as Annas and Veatch appear very dubious about the abilities of ethics committees to steer a clear course. Annas worries about their legalistic tendencies,[4] and Veatch fears they will confuse their role, capitulating to interests other than those of the patients (particularly institutional economic interests); but both share doubts about the adequacy of ethics committees as an institutional response.[5] Moreno, however, while voicing support for committees generally, expresses a deep concern about the process by which ethics committees make decisions, about their trying to work out values in a health care system that is in flux, and about bureaucratic problems inherent in hospital committees.[6] Clinical ethics consultants, in what looks as much like a turf war as anything, claim that ethics committees need to stay out of case review and consultation, leaving that clinically sensitive area to solo practitioners.[7] Lo's often-cited complaint about ethics committees' susceptibility to groupthink is the subtext of many critical articles,[8] as is Blake's insistence that ethics committees lack adequate education and moral authority for their tasks.[9]

Consultation as Primary Mission

At present, it is the committee's involvement in individual treatment decisions that is both its greatest strength (insofar as it is its most interesting activity) and its greatest weakness (insofar as it is so subject to criticism). Ethics committee conferences are inordinately dominated by questions that would not be asked if the committee were not attached to case review. For example: How many people are needed to conduct a case review? Should the committee write in the chart? Should patients be told about case review? Should committees be engaged in case review? From conference questions to journal articles, case review is the focus of virtually all ethics committee controversy and question. It is possible that the future of ethics committees is questionable just because this role is so controversial.[10]

The emphasis in the literature on case review suggests that the future of ethics committees is linked directly to their ability to encourage interest in case review among their colleagues and to conduct case review in an effective and timely manner. In our experience, most committees do relatively little case review (one case per month is on the high side) and worry that this means the committee is a failure. We think there will be a significant increase in case consultation only if it shifts from an optional to a mandatory model.[11]

Physicians currently are not eager to involve themselves with committees. If physicians were to become more willing to seek assistance in their patients' treatment decisions, they and the institutions would, as a practical matter, more likely turn to the individual consultant model. Ethics committees may be less expensive than individual consultants, but they also may be less efficient and, from a chief executive officer's perspective, less reliable. Handing case consultation to the ethics committee involves trusting a somewhat amorphous group rather than a single person with specific and demonstrable credentials. The accountability and credibility of an ethics consultant is simply more obvious because of societal emphasis on expertise and institutional comfort with the placement of individuals, rather than committees, in the hierarchy of authority.

Authority of Ethics Committees

The future of ethics committees as case consultants also is intimately tied to the question of their authority (both moral and practical). To be effective in the consultant role, with its implications of expertise, committees must have some institutional authority. Blake has argued that the source of their moral authority has never been clearly delineated; we would agree with that.[12] We would not agree that that means committees can have no moral authority or role in creating a moral community. However, the nature of their moral authority is not a function of their ethics expertise and thus is not well connected to case consultation insofar as case review appears to require ethics expertise.

Although committees lack moral expertise and thus may not be able to determine what is morally correct in a given treatment dilemma, they can provide a focus and forum for discussions on ethical issues. To the extent that they operate as a closed shop, as if ethics were their province alone (which the consultation model tends to imply), they have no real authority. Many ethics committees feel that they function as "ethics experts" by default, because the institution has delegated this area to them and has established the committee without clearly defining the nature of its authority or responsibility. Doing ethics seriously means institutional and individual change. Too often, the administration or medical staff has ordered up a committee to do education, policy writing, and case review, without any real commitment to any of those activities or without thinking seriously about what an ethics committee doing case consultation really means.

It is possible that future public policy will provide stronger functional (if not moral) authority for ethics committees and their role in case consultation. The experience of Maryland's legislatively mandated ethics committees and of New York's proposed use of ethics committees as surrogate decision makers for patients without surrogates will give us some sense of this. However, in the absence of such broad-scale mandating of ethics committees as case reviewers, committees probably will continue to struggle with their fragile place in the institutional ecology, conducting only a limited number of case consultations. However, their greatest strength will not be their case review work but, rather, their continued commitment to exploring the moral climate of the institution and their willingness to meet regularly and cultivate their interest in bioethics. But the fruits of that cultivation may require a long growing period.

Mission Redefined

Our view of the future of ethics committees is different. If we were to revisit or refine our understanding of the ethics committee mission, we would choose to emphasize its educational aspect, not its consultative one. Like all of medicine, bioethics is an expanding field. Keeping track of new developments in the field and their implications for clinical practice should be the ethics committee's first responsibility (self-education), although not its only one. Just following and understanding these developments may be adequate for a study group that happens to be interested in this kind of material. It is not enough, however, if the group is to be the institution's *ethics committee*. As such, it must offer something to the institution itself.

Furthermore, it should offer something more than a "Mr. Fixit" posture around life-sustaining treatment decisions. If committees were seen in their institutions as a resource for information on ethical perspectives and current ethical debates (rather than as "holders of correct answers"), they could much more easily achieve the second aspect of their mission (educating the community). They also would be more likely to be seen by physicians as potential help rather than as an irrelevance or an interference.

If ethics committees were to understand their primary mission to be education, they also would be able to see that the ethical issues in their institutions do not begin and end in the intensive care unit or the operating room. The emphasis on case consultation has served to limit ethics committees' understanding of ethics in health care as the ethics of the physician–patient relationship rather than the ethics of health care as manifested in the hospital. The ethics of health care institutional practices are much broader and should be of equal and even greater concern to the ethics committee. It would be a sad irony if patients were all treated with exquisite ethical practice when it came to their rights to consent to and refuse life-sustaining treatment, but with ethical indifference during all their other interactions in the hospital, medical center, or long-term care facility. The fact that forgoing life-sustaining treatment decisions was an early focus of bioethics does not mean that the field is defined solely by that issue. Nor should ethics committees define themselves or allow others to define them by that issue.

Even older committees are only now venturing beyond end-of-life treatment decisions. In a thoughtful essay, Fleck has urged committees to become involved in controversial issues such as testing health care professionals for HIV infection.[13] Issues of pain control for patients who are not terminally ill but have chronic pain are beginning to be addressed. If we are sure that issues of addiction are not relevant for the terminally ill patient, can we make the same judgment about addiction and the patient with chronic pain and chronic illness? In a culture that is both enthusiastic about the use of legal drugs and hostile to the use of illegal drugs, how much can/should/must the professional trust the chronically ill patient in assessing need for pain control? These are questions that are of vital importance to many patients and health care professionals, and the field of bioethics has had little to say about them so far. Ethics committees should be thinking about these questions, talking about them, and encouraging others to talk about them to one another.

Some committees in teaching hospitals are beginning to think about the risk to patients when there is poor continuity of care, a particular problem in this setting. What are the ethical issues in structuring patient care in a way that continuity of care is almost certain to suffer? Ethics committees can advocate for patients *and* health care professionals in this area. It means taking a proactive role rather than the reactive role offered by case consultation. Moreover, a positive outcome at this level could lead to the elimination of ethical problems on a broad scale, as opposed to the resolution of a single ethical problem for a single patient.

The ethics committee with well-educated members also should be more concerned, for example, about whether it is represented on other hospitalwide committees than about how many case reviews it has been asked to conduct. Although many originally assumed that the committee's goal was to protect the patient's autonomy, more recent articles have emphasized the ethics committee's duty to ensure responsible health care practice in a broader sense.[14] (This shift in emphasis echoes the arguments in the larger field of bioethics about the proper role of beneficence as opposed to autonomy in the conduct of health care.)

If an ethics committee were to think about its relationship to the practices of the entire hospital, it would understand its work differently. It could see itself as a force for institutional change (rather than for physician change); it could look to the sources of problems in the systems themselves rather than in the individuals who work within those systems. Many of the ethical problems in health care are systemic rather than individual. Responding to those problems requires the committee to see its mission much more broadly. Obviously, its job is not to reform the health care system or even the hospital or long-term care facility of which it is a part. But, within its educational mission, it can lead the way to recognizing the sources of problems and providing those who do have responsibility with different understandings and a stronger voice to bring about change.

This is not to say that ethics committees should be responsible for addressing every ethical issue in the institution. Rather, it is to say that the ethics committee should select the work it chooses to undertake from a broader perspective and a wider range of issues than individual patient care decisions. Such issues might include exploring ways that:

- Physicians and nurses could work together more collegially.
- The hospital could become more user-friendly to patients and families. (For example, why do hospitals in areas with large numbers of Spanish-speaking patients so often have no Spanish language signs? Why are child-oriented pictures in the pediatrics ward hung at the eye level of adults?)
- Everyone could become more reflective about health care resource use.
- Physicians and patients could talk to each other more easily and more clearly.
- Everyone could be more sensitive to helping one another practice universal infection control.
- Patients could feel that they are heard and that their voices are respected in little things, not just in crisis treatment decisions.

For ethics committees to see their mission in this way involves risk taking. It requires courage and confidence because it is a much more amorphous task than doing a case review or writing a policy. Becoming a force for institutional change also means risking failure in a more public and obvious way. These risks can be taken only if the committee has been successful in creating an internal sense of meaning and belonging among its committee members. Ultimately, ethics committees are about the moral nature of being a health care professional, about why it is that health care professionals and their institutions have special obligations and special powers, and about why there is concern about misuse of those powers.

Conclusion

At a time when the American health care system is in transition and there is enormous discouragement about the system as well as the health care professions, the ethics committee provides a place in which the values and meaning of health care are acknowledged, discussed, and renewed—the very reason why people join the committee. The authors are repeatedly struck by the devotion of most ethics committee members and their concern for the committee's well-being and future. The authors have not noticed this phenomenon in other health care institutional committees. (A corporate lawyer visiting a monthly ethics and literature seminar organized by ethics committee members from several hospitals noted, with surprise, "I don't know any lawyers anywhere doing this kind of thing!") There is something about the idea of the ethics committee that goes deeply to the heart of many health care professionals. Perhaps it is because, as the health care institution has increasingly focused on its business concerns, the workplace has felt increasingly barren of values. Those values continue to be affirmed in ethics committees and their members are grateful for that.

However, the ethics committee of the future will need to do more than affirm those values. It will need to show where the institution has lost or neglected them and how they can be restored or reaffirmed in creative and even lighthearted ways. Health care institutions have been forced to change in recent years and will change more in the coming ones. In the process of making these changes, long-standing values often have inadvertently been neglected. It can be the job of ethics committees—working in their institution, with ethics committees from other institutions, within networks, and with their community—now and in the future to remind their institutions what those values are and why they are still important.

Notes and References

1. Rothman, D. *Strangers at the Bedside.* New York City: Basic Books, 1991.

2. For a discussion of various attempts to mandate ethics committees, see: Hoffman, D. E. Regulating ethics committees in health care institutions—is it time? *Maryland Law Review* 50(3):746–97, 1991.

3. See, for example, Wolf, S. M. Ethics committees and due process. *Maryland Law Review* 50(3):798–858, 1991; and Wolf, S. M. Due process in ethics committee case review. *HEC Forum* 4(2):83–96, 1992.

4. Annas, G. Ethics committees: from ethical comfort to ethical cover. *Hastings Center Report* 21(3):18–21, 1991.

5. Veatch, R. M. The ethics of institutional committees. In: R. E. Cranford and A. E. Doudera, Jr., editors. *Institutional Ethics Committees and Health Care Decision Making.* Ann Arbor, MI: Health Administration Press, 1984, pp. 35–50.

6. Moreno, J. Ethics committees: proceed with caution. *Maryland Law Review* 50(3):895–903, 1991.

7. Agich, F. J., and Youngner, S. J. For experts only? Access to hospital ethics committees. *Hastings Center Report* 21(5):17–25, 1991; and LaPuma, J., and Toulmin, S. Ethics consultants and ethics committees. *Archives of Internal Medicine* 149(5):1109–12, 1989.

8. Lo, B. Behind closed doors: promise and pitfalls of ethics committees. *New England Journal of Medicine* 317(1):46–50, 1987; and Blake, D. The irony of the ethics committee. *Ethical Currents* 17:5, 7, 1988.

9. Blake, D. The hospital ethics committee and moral authority. *HEC Forum* 4(5):6–8, 1992.

10. Povar, G. J. Evaluating ethics committees: what do we mean by success? *Maryland Law Review* 50(3):904–19, 1991; Griener, G. G., and Storch, J. L. Hospital ethics committees: problems in evaluation. *HEC Forum* 4(1):5–8, 1992; and Van Allen, E., Moldow, D. G., and Cranford, R. Evaluating ethics committees. *Hastings Center Report* 19(5):23–24, 1989.

11. Robertson, J. A. Committees as decision makers: alternative structures and responsibilities. In: R. E. Cranford and A. E. Doudera, editors. *Institutional Ethics Committees and Health Care Decision Making.* Ann Arbor, MI: Health Administration Press, 1984, pp. 85–95.

12. Blake, The hospital ethics committee and moral authority.

13. Fleck, L. HIV-infected health professionals: what to do? *Ethics-in-Formation* 3(6):1–2, 1991.

14. Agich and Youngner.

Additional Books of Interest

Making Choices: Ethics Issues for Health Care Professionals
edited by Emily Friedman

". . . a sturdy collection of vintage and recent papers that should be familiar—and of continuing use—to all who confront troublesome issues . . . Ms. Friedman and the American Hospital Association have performed a superb service in compiling this collection of ethically relevant gems."

Richard S. Scott, M.D., J.D., in *New England Journal of Medicine*

Making Choices: Ethics Issues for Health Care Professionals brings together 28 original and landmark articles that present perspectives on both the issues and the possible courses of action. The book presents numerous points of view that cover 30 years in the field of hospital ethics and provide lessons from the past as well as guidance for the future.
1986. 246 pages, 14 tables, 3 figures.
ISBN 0-939450-77-1
Catalog No. E99-025100
$29.95 (AHA members, $24.00)

Handbook for Hospital Ethics Committees
by Judith Wilson Ross, with Sister Corrine Bayley, Vicki Michel, and Deborah Pugh

". . . useful to those involved in ethically sound medical decision making . . . a lucid, comprehensible addition to the growing literature concerned with the quality of ethical analysis."

Marshall B. Kapp, Department of Medicine in Society, Wright State University School of Medicine in *Journal of Gerontology*

Handbook for Hospital Ethics Committees examines the nature and purpose of ethics committees and provides practical suggestions for committee members in defining their roles and responsibilities.
1986. 176 pages, bibliography, index.
ISBN 0-939450-96-8
Catalog No. E99-025101
$28.75 (AHA members, $23.00)

Choices and Conflict: Explorations in Health Care Ethics
edited by Emily Friedman

"*Choices and Conflict* is excellent. It contains a broader diversity of health care systems issues than most collections, including articles from the field of public health that have been too long ignored. I strongly recommend it."

Daniel E. Beauchamp, Professor, School of Public Health, Department of Health Policy and Management, University of Albany, New York

This companion volume to *Making Choices* provides the most advanced thinking on ethics issues for the health care professional. With a foreword by George D. Lundberg, M.D., editor of the *Journal of the American Medical Association,* the book contains 22 landmark and 6 original articles written by leading health care attorneys, ethicists, sociologists, physicians, and nurses.

Important and timely topics, such as patient rights issues (AIDS patients' access to care, patient autonomy, right-to-die issues), rising costs (rationing issues, technology), and much more are addressed.
1992. 221 pages.
ISBN 1-55648-082-2
Catalog No. E99-025105
$42.00 (AHA members, $32.00)